RHETORIC, MEDICINE, AND THE WOMAN WRITER, 1600–1700

How did physicians come to dominate the medical profession? Lyn Bennett challenges the seemingly self-evident belief that scientific competence accounts for physicians' dominance. Instead, she argues that the whole enterprise of learned medicine was, in large measure, facilitated by an intensely classical education that included extensive training in rhetoric, and that this rhetorical training is ultimately responsible for the achievement of professional dominance. Bennett examines previously unexplored connections among writers and genres as well as competing livelihoods and classes. Engaging the histories of rhetoric, medicine, literature, and culture throughout, she goes on to focus specifically on the work of women who professed as well as practiced medicine. Pointing to some of the ways women's writing shapes realities of body, mind, and spirit as it negotiates social, cultural, and professional ideologies of gender, this book offers an important corrective to some long-held beliefs about women's role in early modern discourse.

LYN BENNETT is an associate professor of English at Dalhousie University, Nova Scotia. Her interest in rhetoric, writing, and medicine informs her teaching as well as her research. She is the author of *Women Writing of Divinest Things: Rhetoric in the Poetry of Pembroke, Wroth, and Lanyer* (2004), and her work also appears in publications as diverse as *Christianity and Literature, Genre,* and the *Journal of Medical Humanities*.

RHETORIC, MEDICINE, AND THE WOMAN WRITER, 1600–1700

LYN BENNETT

Dalhousie University

CAMBRIDGE
UNIVERSITY PRESS

CAMBRIDGE
UNIVERSITY PRESS

University Printing House, Cambridge CB2 8BS, United Kingdom

One Liberty Plaza, 20th Floor, New York, NY 10006, USA

477 Williamstown Road, Port Melbourne, VIC 3207, Australia

314–321, 3rd Floor, Plot 3, Splendor Forum, Jasola District Centre, New Delhi – 110025, India

79 Anson Road, #06-04/06, Singapore 079906

Cambridge University Press is part of the University of Cambridge.

It furthers the University's mission by disseminating knowledge in the pursuit of education, learning, and research at the highest international levels of excellence.

www.cambridge.org
Information on this title: www.cambridge.org/9781108425193
DOI: 10.1017/9781108348218

First published 2018

Printed in the United Kingdom by Clays, St Ives plc

A catalogue record for this publication is available from the British Library.

ISBN 978-1-108-42519-3 Hardback

For all the sisters making their way in a man's world.

Contents

Preface

There is no denying the significance of early modern medicine to the profession we know today. Yet medical historians would agree that the answer to how a small group of rather disengaged healers evolved to become the "prestigious" and "supremely well-entrenched" profession Roy Porter identifies lies only in part with increasing success in alleviating suffering and saving lives ("The Patient's View" 175). Treatment may have become at least perceptually more effective with the scientific turn of a "new" medicine whose rise, Eliot Freidson points out, coincided with growing reliance on "careful observation" through the seventeenth and eighteenth centuries (15), yet the inflection of a once-overwhelmingly theoretical epistemology with the practical and applied does not tell the whole story. It may be true that, despite "all their intellectual pretensions," as Mark Jenner and Patrick Wallis suggest, "learned physicians did not command any real degree of cultural authority until the nineteenth century" (2), but it is equally true that it took discursive shape in the seventeenth, facilitated in large measure by the classical education that became less important to the physicians' self-fashioning even as it enabled the "emergence" of what Margaret Pelling and Charles Webster identify as "a university-educated elite at the head of the nascent medical profession" (235).

The seventeenth-century physician thus "known for his sensitive control of the Latin tongue" was not, however, necessarily also "respected for his wide acquaintance with the classics" or the "much else" James L. Axtell as recently as 1970 was persuaded to declare. Given that early modern physicians were also subjects of suspicion and ridicule, the esteem Axtell confers on a profession perhaps more beleaguered than respected does suggest that our "fascination with medicine," as Pelling proposes, is at least in part inspired by its "late and dramatic change from comparatively humble origins." Persuading even retrospective concession to their escalating "demands for respect and rewards," the self-fashioning enterprise of those

Lucinda Beier styles as "Foremost among medical propagandists" (2) may have been equally well served by the writing of a history that, Pelling proposes, has granted comparatively "little critical attention" to the nascent emergence of the profession we know today ("Trade or Profession" 230–31).[1] Enabled by tools as effective as those of "the natural philosophers' own rhetorical kitbag," the terms and tenets that gave voice to their professionalizing enterprise may, Juliet Cummins and David Burchell note, "seem self-evident to us" (2), but the physicians' efforts could not have succeeded if not for the intensity and scope of an education that made their medical practice no more effective but did grant them persuasive advantage over rivals often better equipped for healing success.

Waged in what Beier dubs a "two-pronged campaign" that worked "to create a favourable image for licensed healers" while aiming "to destroy the reputation and practices" of the unlicensed (33), the means of the physicians' rise in what was once a diverse "medical marketplace" is a story already well told.[2] As much as historians have done to reveal the workings

[1] According to Pelling, it remains an open question whether seventeenth-century medicine is the archetype of modern professions, hence stable and definable, or whether it remains "a larger field, more various, less controlled, and more fragmented" than such a definition allows ("Trade or Profession" 258). Keith M. MacDonald, on the other hand, argues that "the professions started to appear in their present form contemporaneously with modern capitalist industrial society." Yet it is nevertheless clear that the early modern physicians shared with the modern what MacDonald defines as "the professional project," which "has as its objectives the securing, enhancement and maintenance of the social and economic standing of its members, and thus the achievement of a relative advantage in the structure of inequality" (36). At the same time, MacDonald recognizes the difficulty in defining "profession" to serve as anything more than "a kind of shorthand" instead of "a closely defined technical term" and admits that "'professional' and similar terms have a wide range of uses in everyday speech" that are most often "value-laden" (1). Jan Goldstein agrees establishing "a suitable definition has produced disagreement among sociologists," who nevertheless seem to concur on "a list of the formal attributes" indicating "at least some degree of sociological consensus" and including

> (1) a body of esoteric knowledge, mastery of which is the indispensable qualification for practice of the profession; (2) monopoly – that is, recognition of the exclusive competence of the profession in the domain to which its body of knowledge refers; (3) autonomy, or control by the profession over its work, including who can legitimately do that work and how the work should be done; and (4) a service ideal – that is, a commitment or ethical imperative to place the welfare of the public or of the individual client above the self-interest of the practitioner (174–75).

There is no question that the seventeenth-century physicians fashioned themselves as masters of "a body of esoteric knowledge," that they aimed to control the profession's work, most obviously through the London College, and that they voiced a "service ideal." Though the physicians' monopoly was far from clear at the beginning of the seventeenth century, the profession that emerged by the end was predicated on the "the body of knowledge" Goldstein describes as "the absolutely necessary" of those "four attributes" that was either "deliberately stressed or simply taken for granted" (175). It seems as well that the specialized knowledge once so clearly stressed worked to become largely "taken for granted" (175); there is also little question that the discourse of learned medicine was as "value-laden" as the latter-day usages MacDonald attributes to the term "profession."

[2] Mark S. R. Jenner and Patrick Wallis note that there has been subsequent debate over the term "medical marketplace," overuse perhaps rendering the concept less meaningful and as "overdue for revision" as Pelling claims (qtd in Jenner and Wallis 2). The term is useful here, however, in describing

of early modern medicine, however, "The analytical techniques honed by literary scholars are," as Monica Green points out, also "important tools in excavating the shifting meanings and uses of medical texts" (11) and, I would add, they are tools that prove equally useful in pointing to some of the ways the physicians negotiated their dominion over practitioners often better equipped for healing success. The product of a professionalizing campaign so successful that Freidson's landmark study of medicine as the "sociology of applied knowledge" proceeds from the assumption "that if anything 'is' a profession, it is contemporary medicine" (4), the physicians' rise was enabled also by extensive training in the rhetorical art so integral to the early modern culture in which they lived and worked. Though the physicians' appeals cannot, of course, be utterly divorced from the epistemological and applied, my focus is not on the *what* but the *how* of what the physicians professed and the ways in which their rhetoric intersects with discourses religious, popular, and literary.

Given that the means to describe "what for centuries had remained below the threshold of the visible and the expressible" emerged only in the nineteenth, the clinical gaze that worked to forge "A new alliance" between "words and things" was, as Michel Foucault explains, unavailable to earlier physicians, whose limited access to the internal body necessitated a heavier reliance on the word. What would later become defined by the "empirical vigilance" Foucault describes as "receptive only to the evidence of visible contents" was hitherto an epistemology less trustful of the visible and more reliant on the speculative. Having reasoned its way into faith, then, the language of medicine could not help but retain "the stigmatas of its historical origin" manifest in "an exegesis" inevitably harkening back "to the Word of God" in a culture as religious as it was rhetorical. As Foucault's words suggest, the means of medicine's "late and dramatic change" cannot be separated from discourses that, despite the emergence of the new science and the oft-invoked Cartesian divide, were inflected by the uncertainty of a language that, as Foucault says, is always and ultimately "ever secret" and "ever beyond itself." Fashioned through the "theories and old systems" that may have made "clinical *experience* possible" (Foucault, Intro.), the rhetoric of early modern medicine could not transcend the religious any more than it could utterly refute the practical medicine to which the learned physicians lay increasing claim, and it equally resists the order we may seek in our own attempts to impose shape on that which is not easily defined.

a medical context that included myriad practitioners beyond the licensed physicians, surgeons, and apothecaries.

Yet, as Elizabeth Lane Furdell and others have shown, the complex relations of print, medicine, and professional competition unique to the seventeenth century present an especially rich matrix for examining the complex process of a profession coming into being. What that matrix suggests is that the learned physicians' high degree of literacy and extensive knowledge of rhetoric cannot in themselves account for the success of a campaign that saw medicine emerge as "the archetypal profession," as Gordon Horobin reminds us, only "by common assent" (90). The physicians were not alone in fashioning what would become exceptional only by virtue of a "*social* process" that, notes Jan Goldstein, is as crucial as an "*intellectual* core" (175) to any profession's making. Pointing to that which makes the medicine's rise, like natural philosophy's, also "seem a little less natural and inevitable" (Cummins and Burchell 2), this study focuses on a rhetoric substantively and formally recognizable yet variously inflected as it does its persuasive work. Given that rhetorical analysis, as David Harley argues, can also reveal some of the "connections between the larger social constructions" in which "medical beliefs and elaborated theories" operate ("Social Construction" 435), the examination that follows also considers how the beliefs and theories of learned medicine are corroborated, elaborated, and challenged in the work of writers who were not physicians.

Focusing especially on the women from whom the physicians insistently sought to distinguish themselves, what follows does much to confirm Monica Green's claim that "the suppression of women's authority in the male spheres of literate, professionalized medicine was nearly absolute." As much as their hands-on counterparts', the rhetoric even of those who wrote about but did not actively practice healing equally suggests that women were indeed "never completely passive in the face of masculine dominance" (Green 290). Though the most disdained of the many alternative healers the physicians complained about as well as their most vilified patients, women of varying classes and circumstances engaged and sometimes overtly challenged medicine's dominant discourse, and they did so in works devotional and literary as well as medical. Yet it is telling of the extent to which the authority of the male sphere penetrated all of early modern culture that, even in resisting their discursive exclusion from the healing and rhetorical arts to which they could lay just claim, women could not help but facilitate the physicians' professionalizing enterprise even as they strove to claim a social and cultural authority of their own.

Acknowledgments

This project could not have been completed without the help of a Social Sciences and Humanities Research Council of Canada Research Grant, and I am thankful for SSHRC's generous support over the years. Thanks are also owed to the *Journal of Medical Humanities*, in which parts of Chapter 4 originally appeared, and to the reviewer whose helpful comments made for a better essay. My colleagues and my Faculty at Dalhousie University have facilitated my research with sabbatical leaves and their cheerful willingness to engage with work long in progress. For their unfailing support and encouragement, I am grateful. Halifax's Medieval and Early Modern Reading Group provided useful feedback on Chapter 1, and thanks are owed to John Baxter, Christina Luckyj, Krista Kesselring, and Tim Stretton for their thoughtful input. To John Baxter and to the late Peter Medway I am indebted for all they have done to inspire and shape my thinking in all things rhetorical. Feedback on numerous conference presentations has been unfailingly encouraging and helpful, and I owe a debt of gratitude to the many organizers, presenters, and attendees for their contributions to the final product. I am especially grateful to have shared the company of Stephen Pender, Edith Snook, and Jennifer Richards, the finest of scholars whose example never fails to inspire. Graduate students in my seminar on early modern illness and writing have fertilized my thinking in a number of ways over the past several years, and I owe much to their enthusiasm, intelligence, and fresh perspectives. Of them, special thanks are due to Adam Bowes, who proved a diligent and imaginative research assistant, and whose hard work steered me toward some texts that both complicated and refined my thinking. The fruits of his labour appear throughout. The deepest of thanks are, of course, owed to the rigorous and capable editors of Cambridge University Press, and to the reviewers of the original and revised manuscripts, whose generosity and knowledge improved my work immensely.

This book could not have been written without the support of family and friends. I am most grateful to Eve, Russell, and Emily Court for understanding why I'm sometimes unavailable even when physically present, and to Trevor Ross for his sage advice as well as everything he does to ease the demands of a busy life. My Ottawa siblings, Natalie and Rob, and their partners, Paul and Sandy, have generously shared a place to recharge and have some fun, while sister Sue has long provided merriment at home. Mary Lou Martin, Laura Methot, and Lesley Williams have offered loving and supportive friendship and they, along with the city of New Orleans, are owed special thanks. That Laura also generously read and commented on an earlier version of this book deserves special mention, not only for her enthusiasm but also for her understanding that one need not be a humanist to appreciate the humanities. Finally, much love and gratitude are owed to Russ and Myrna, the ever-loyal parents who have long been my biggest fans.

Introduction
"Their Plausible Rhetorick"

> 'Tis unspeakable how these Galenists have imposed upon credulous men, how by their plausible Rhetorick they have allured them, and made the people willingly to resign their Lives up to their Judgements, notwithstanding all those sad presidents lively represented to their eyes. What fair pretences have they made use of to gull them into their Physick? What a supercillious command have they had over their obsequious Apothecary, to speak for them, to lye for them; yea, and to do some things for them, to the hazard of his Soul; being forced to maintain, and sometimes to own all their miscarriages, misdemeanours, and gross aberrations in Physick, or else he, his wife and children must bite on the bridle. These are they that have infused into the people abominable vulgar Errors in Physick, which neither Doctor Primerose, Doctor Browne, nor a thousand like them, are able by the best of Rhetorick or Logick to eradicate.
>
> George Thomson, *Galeno-pale* (1665)

Disputing the London College, chemical physician George Thomson faults those who persuade patients "willingly to resign their Lives up to their Judgements" while denying the many "miscarriages, misdemeanours, and gross aberrations in Physick." The "fair pretences" of "these Galenists," Thomson argues, cannot be eradicated by even "the best of Rhetorick or Logick" (15). A disciple of van Helmont who saw little value in Galenism, Thomson challenged College physician Nathaniel Hodges to put "their two methods of practice to a trial" with the goal of proving once and for all, explains Harold Cook, that "the learned physicians were the truly illegitimate practitioners" (*Medical Regime* 160). Thomson's aim was, of course, to champion his chemical practice over the bookish ways of a College that comprised physicians whose success owed more to rhetorical effect than healing efficacy. In opposing unlicensed practitioners and recruiting James Primrose and Sir Thomas Browne to his persuasive ends, however, Thomson also takes the learned physicians' part in making his case. Thus fashioning distinctions nebulous at best and spurious at worst, Thomson's own rhetoric suggests something of how early modern medicine worked to shape, distinguish, and uphold disciplinary *différance*. Whether serving the proponents of change or the Galenist old guard, and regardless of whether the debate centred on the differences among physicians or between physicians and all other kinds of practitioners, such a "plausible Rhetoricke" worked to the professionalizing ends of those who would eventually claim the lion's share of medical practice.[1]

The physicians' plausible mode of persuasion reveals much about how the success of what was once the most esoteric, detached, and impractical of medicine's many branches was enabled by the discursive fashioning of a profession prestigious in its distinction from other professions, from the hands-on practices of medical rivals, and from the patients it professed to treat. Persuasive to the extent that the physicians' self-fashioning enterprise was facilitated as much as challenged in the texts of rival, dissenting, and lay writers, medicine's oft-conflicted rhetoric did much also to shape the texts of women who took up topics of illness and healing. We cannot, of course, recognize the import of women's participation in a given culture without some understanding of what that culture entails. I therefore offer this study in two parts. Attending to a rhetoric that foregrounds the practitioner and purports to address a rival or popular audience, each of the three chapters that Part I comprises takes up a particular site of contention in examining learned medicine's self-fashioning and revealing some of the ways alternative writers resist and support the physicians' professionalizing campaign. The analysis that follows thus begins in Chapter 1 by considering the physicians' debate with those clerics who deigned to practise medicine, focuses in Chapter 2 on their resistance to the many alternative healers with whom the physicians vied, and concludes in Chapter 3 by examining the discursive fashioning of the patients on whose aquiescence medical authority depended.

In their self-fashioning aims, the physicians who are the focus of Chapter 1 prove particularly intent on articulating what David Harley describes as a more "general distaste" for any mingling of "the two separate

[1] Galenic thinking may not have been as thoroughly entrenched as the physicians would have us believe: "Even among physicians," Oswei Temkin notes, "its claim to universality was rarely heeded" (171). Yet it is also true that Galenism continued to inflect medical thinking and practice well into the eighteenth century, and it influenced much more than Renaissance medicine. Inflecting early modern thinking in various and broad ways, "Galenism," Temkin argues, was in actuality "a general intellectual phenomenon restricted to neither medicine nor philosophy, to neither one nation nor one culture" (192). Despite some insistence to the contrary, there were few medical practitioners in the seventeenth century who were not influenced by Galen.

vocations of clergyman and physician" ("Calvinist Critique" 368). In a context where bodily and spiritual healing were never entirely separable, however, the physicians's arguments relied also on the rhetoric of religion, its necessity perhaps undeniable in any challenge to the university-educated clerics whose divinely ordained mandate was claimed also by the physicians.[2] Yet discursive inclusion went only one way, and the physicians show no qualms about denying their clerical competition the right to participate in their own. Thus enacting the "paradox of distinctiveness and openness" Andrew Wear finds more specifically in the protection and dissemination of medical knowledge ("Popularization" 19), the physicians' professionalizing rhetoric attests to its conflicting impulses in varied and complex arguments that cannot finally uphold the distinctions they aim to assert. Their "plausible Rhetoricke" may have served their self-fashioning aims, but the physicians' attempts to define a discipline denied to others were also compromised by the language they deployed.

As Galenism increasingly gave way to what Richard Sugg describes as "a legitimate pluralism of competing beliefs" (27), the physicians also grew loud in their objections to the many nonclerical rivals considered in Chapter 2. Disputing alternative healers who, as Lucinda Beier points out, represented "the vast majority of people practicing medicine" and therefore threatening in numbers alone (19), the physicians worked to discredit not only the disdained "petticoat" doctors and despised "empirics," but also the less-educated surgeon and "obsequious Apothecary" chastised even by the anti-Galenist Thomson (15). Drawing authority from the "theoretical skill" that, says Cook, defined theirs "as a philosophy of health" (*Medical Regime* 62–63), the physicians championed their superior education while decrying the practical orientation of rivals whose experiential epistemology stood in oft-professed opposition to their own. Conflated to an undifferentiated body of error against which learned medicine could posit its distinctiveness, myriad alternative practitioners serve as the discursive foil to a profession increasingly open to adopting the very practices it decried. The profession of medicine, in other words, may have insistently aligned

[2] Beier argues that because "there was no consensus in the general population that licensed healers were the sole authorities in medical matters," there was also "no medical profession in seventeenth-century England." Though it is true that "the creation of a profession requires such a consensus" (4–5), Beier's point may have more to do with degree than kind. It is arguable as well that there was consensus among at least some members of the populace that worked to buttress the physicians' authority, thus colluding in the professional self-fashioning of physicians who, says Cook, "self-consciously used the word 'profession' with regard to themselves and to no other medical practitioners" ("Good Advice" 4).

itself with theory and philosophy, but its self-fashioning efforts depended also on the practical and rhetorical arts it so often disclaimed.

Yet the openness and distinctiveness that are a hallmark of learned medicine's quarrel with the clergy and other medical practitioners becomes mere distinction when treating of the subjects who are the focus of Chapter 3. Wielding their "plausible Rhetorick" to broadly subjugating effect, the physicians assert dominion over all patients but prove particularly intent on instilling obedience in those who are female. Confirming physician Andrew Boorde's belief that the need for a "placable" subject is met by the necessary command of "a rethorick or an eloquent tongue" ("The Preface" n. pag.), however, the persuasive lengths the physicians are willing to go also suggest an authority hard won over patients who were subjects in more ways than one. Not only must physicians read both visually and verbally from texts proffered by those who must to some extent control them, patient autonomy and agency cannot be utterly denied in a context where the faculties of mind, body, and spirit are as symbiotic as they are identifiable. Deploying whatever means available to ensure compliance, the physicians could not relegate even the female patient to a merely submissive body any more than they could wholly deny the interconnection of medical and religious ways of knowing that were ever linked with rhetoric.

Building on the groundwork laid in Part I, the three chapters of Part II consider some of the ways the rhetoric of early modern medicine makes itself known in the discourse of women who took up topics of illness and healing. That rhetoric, medicine, and religion are parallel and sometimes interdependent endeavours becomes especially clear in light of the culturally understood advantages of illness considered in Chapter 4. Deploying language to cope with as well as express affliction, women who write about illness and healing tend to predicate their authority on the religious discourse to which every believer could lay rightful claim. Yet, given the many and widespread injunctions against female speech as well as entrenched beliefs about myriad bodily afflictions thought to inflict the feminine mind, negotiating terms from which to speak credibly also proves more urgent for women who write about, through, or from illness. Though very much inflected by the gendered expectations of discourses religious and medical, the rhetoric of women who write of illness yet shares with that of the physicians and the physician-clerics the overarching primacy of its self-fashioning and self-authorizing aims.

Further giving the lie to physician John Sadler's belief that women must be addressed so as not "to confound your understandings with a more Rhetoricall discourse" ("The Epistle Dedicatory" n. pag.), Chapter 5 suggests that at least some women wrote to establish their place in the histories of rhetoric and of the professions. Discernible in the work of those from different decades, origins, and circumstances, women's engagement with the discourse of learned medicine further explains the physicians' desire to exclude others from the art so crucial to their own success. Revealing much about their threatening potential, women who engage learned medicine prove themselves knowing rhetors in assuming a subject position very different from the explicitly devotional orientation of their afflicted counterparts. Confirming that the boundaries of medical discourse and the profession it aimed to define were more open and fluid than the physicians' rhetoric admits, women also assert the distinctiveness of the discourse community into which they inscribe their own belonging. Sometimes complicit with even when resisting its insistently distinguishing rhetoric, women who write about learned medicine thus understand as well as any physician that language artfully used is crucial to establishing and maintaining the bounds of any profession.

Women's medical writing was not only shaped but also appropriated by men. Though elsewhere insisting that women's healing practices do little good at best and grievous harm at worst, the male editors and publishers considered in Chapter 6 are not reticent about laying claim to feminine knowledge in disseminating the remedy collections that proved key to medicine's popularization. More open in intent yet dependent in large measure on the domestic work of women, the mediating rhetoric of the remedy books tends to ignore or occlude the origins of the knowledge they present, and women are therefore denied meaningful participation in its making. Thus working both to assimilate and deny the efforts of those they frequently derided but, as Beier puts it, from whom they "happily accepted medical recipes" (43), those who lay claim to domestic knowledge work either to discredit women's part in its making or to abstract it so far from practical application that their efforts become inconsequential. Subject to a rhetoric forceful enough to insinuate itself even into discourses aiming to resist it, the women claiming authorship whose works are considered later in the chapter can be seen also to collude with male authority in claiming legitimacy for their own offerings.

It seems, then, that the more knowledgeable and confident a woman author, the more likely she would be to participate in giving voice and credence to learned medicine's self-fashioning. In taking on the terms of what they sometimes aimed to redress, women who wrote as sufferers and healers were in some ways as invested in upholding dominant authority as those men who lay untroubled claim to women's healing knowledge. What their engagement suggests, however, is not that early modern women conceded unwittingly to cultural demands but that they too participated in, and therefore helped also to fashion, a rhetoric most often construed as the product and province of men. Contrary to what we might expect from the gender most often relegated to the tending of household business, women who wrote about illness and recovery, both those who practised healing and those who did not, thus enacted early modern medicine's paradox of "distinctiveness and openness" as they negotiated or aligned themselves with a range of medical, professional, and social groups as well as epistemological and disciplinary allegiances. Ultimately, rhetorical analyses of their debates suggest that the terms of the seventeenth century's medical rivalry offered to an array of writers a wealth of persuasive resources as well as points of contention that, at least in part, inspired and enabled their voices in dynamic, complex, and sometimes contradictory ways.

PART I

Rhetoric and Medicine

CHAPTER 1

"Another Mans Profession"
Physicians and Clerics

In 1673, the self-styled John Smith, Gent. published *The Mysterie of Rhetorick Unveil'd*, proclaiming on its title page to be "Eminently delightful and profitable for young Scholars, and others of all sorts, enabling them to discern and imitate the Elegancy in any Author they read, *&c.*" Offering training appropriate for "all sorts" as well as scholars, Smith understands rhetoric's broad application and appeal. This is not to say, however, that he does not also understand rhetoric as a discipline unto itself; though useful to all, rhetoric was thought best taught and theorized about by rhetoricians. Smith, however, probes their professional domain in "The Author to the Reader," where he lays claim to the rhetorician's subject:

> Were it absolutely necessary for him that would write of Eloquence to be perfectly eloquent, I would easily confess my self too rash in this enterprise: But having seen often those treat knowingly of painting that never held Pencil, and *Cicero* remarking the *Aratus*, by the common consent of learned men, wrote excellently of the Heavens & Stars, though he was no noted Astronomer; I'm encourag'd to say, why then may not I too discourse of Eloquence without being an Oratour? (Sig. $A4_r$)

Smith's question is a rhetorical one, an *erotema* whose implied answer is that he may indeed "treat knowingly" of rhetoric, just as those of his proffered *exempla* have treated of art or astronomy even when lacking formal training or practical experience.

Smith may, however, understand his transgression more than he admits. Anticipating objections to an undertaking "too rash" for those less than "perfectly eloquent," Smith's self-refuting *procatalepsis* in itself suggests as much. Evincing its author's awareness of a disciplinary intrusion incompatible with his enterprise, *The Mysterie of Rhetorick Unveil'd* was published late in a century in which professional boundaries were becoming more firmly defined, and Smith therefore more urgently compelled to acknowledge the limits of his expertise.[1] Accordingly, he admits that those "able to set down the rules and laws which ought to be observed in speech or style, may notwithstanding find himself defective in the application." Confessing that he may be able to tell but cannot show, however, Smith excuses his shortcomings as a rhetor but plays the rhetorician, insisting that the rulemaker can offer "that to others, which he hath not himself" (Sig. $A4_v$). Hence "this treatise indeed may not so properly be termed a Direction to the Art of Rhetorique" but "a Key to unlock and lay open those abstruse difficulties which the Tropes and Figures have hither to, not only been masked with, but lock'd up under." Smith's is not a modest position, for in claiming a capacity to teach but not necessarily do, he asserts a level of command over his subject higher than those who write mere "Direction." Taking the part of theory over *praxis*, Smith thus likens himself to "*Galen*, the great Master of Physick," who was able to write "so learnedly of every part of that Science" though "little seen in the Practick" (Sig. $A4_r$).[2] Granted, Smith aims to address those who may be "altogether unacquainted with the *Greek* tongue, and have not directed their studies to that subject," but makes clear that he is able to do so not only because he shares the rhetoricians' linguistic knowledge but can also explicate some "abstruse difficulties" in ways they have not. Aligning his work with that of the higher-order professional and not the hands-on practitioner, Smith shares with the early modern and ancient physician an ethos fashioned in contrast with a sometimes only implied but always present other.[3]

Sharing also what Stephen Pender describes as rhetoric's "forays into the probable" ("Medicine and Rhetoric" 36), the profession that is both science

1 Freidson defines a profession as "distinct from other occupations in that it has been given the right to control its work" (71); he would, however, also argue that medicine is the occupation most readily identifiable as a "profession" (4).

2 Smith extends the relevance of the merely theoretical to warcraft as well, arguing, "Nor are those that discourse best of the embatttailing Armies, & differencing Military functions, always the best Warriers, or the most daring" (Sig. $A4_r$–$A4_v$).

3 Representing one of the three professions (divinity, law, and medicine) surviving from the Middle Ages, the physicians fashioned theirs over against a medical other by emphasizing the lengthy education necessary to "exercise good judgment and advice" that, Cook argues, could not result solely from knowledge but "had to be tempered with inner discipline and deep consideration" to shape the "physician of good character" ("Good Advice" 4). More recent shifts in sociological paradigms have, Keith MacDonald explains, seen the adoption of an "action-based theory" that "played an important role in the functionalist depiction of modern society" where "work and occupations in general were ethically neutral" while "the professions were seen as being ethically positive" and thus "embodiments of the 'central values' of the society" (xi). The exercise of "good judgment and advice," I would argue, was equally an action, and it was an action crucial to fashioning of the early modern professional's ethos.

and art has long been allied with that of using language to persuade.[4] Echoing the grudging recognition of Plato's ever-suspicious Socrates that "medicine has to define the nature of the body and rhetoric of the soul" (49), Thomas Wilson confirms as much in his 1560 *Art of Rhetoric*, where he recognizes persuasion's importance to body and soul: it is through the right use and application of language, he affirms, that "the weak would be comforted" and the passions "brought under the obedience of reason" (102).[5] Later, physician Sir Thomas Browne would write in his *Religio Medici* of his epiphanic recognition of rhetoric's epistemological force: "That we are the breath and similitude of God, it is indisputable," Browne proclaims, "but to call ourselves a microcosm, or little world, I thought it only a pleasant trope of rhetorick, till my near judgment and second thoughts told me there was a real truth therein" (*Religio* 24: part 1, sec. 34). Even for the scientifically oriented Browne, rhetoric enables the understanding of a mind inseparable from body and soul. Simultaneously invoking or at least alluding to the disciplines of rhetoric, medicine, and religion, Wilson and Browne offer a particularly salient illustration of the inevitable interconnection of three distinct yet ever-intersecting disciplines.

Rhetoric became even more valuable to the physicians as their rivals in strength and number grew in tandem with demand.[6] Fuelled by a public increasingly interested in and knowledgeable about health care, the medical-professional contest between the physicians and other

[4] Despite Plato's early recognition of rhetoric's significance to medicine, the art of using language well has been "sorely neglected," says Stephen Pender, as an "aspect of medical thought from antiquity through to the early modern period" ("Medicine and Rhetoric" 41), even though, as David Harley remarks, "Rhetoric has always been even more central to medicine than it is to the natural sciences" ("Social Construction" 421). Medicine's reliance on rhetoric also had much to do with the physicians' protectionist agenda. Unlike their medical counterparts, emerging scientists preferred to share what they discovered; as Barbara J. Shapiro once pointed out, the ideas of the new science were not "the exclusive possession of a small or isolated scientific community," and "scientists did not think of themselves as a closed professional community"; rather, "most scientific publications were directed to the general reading public," and "writers like Bacon and Galileo displayed an almost missionary zeal to spread the faith of the new science" (732–33).

[5] That rhetoric serves "in private troubles" as well as "common miseries" (102) Wilson further affirms. Building likewise "on classical precedent," Stephen Pender notes, George Puttenham's 1589 *Arte of English Poesie* posits even death as "susceptible to poetic and rhetorical cure," and therefore urges "poets to 'play' physicians" in applying their persuasive " 'medicine to the ordinary sicknes of mankind' " ("Imagination" 72). Language's curative possibilities have more recently been addressed in John Coulehan's meaning-centred model of illness and Brian Stock's reintegrated body, mind, and spirit, studies that reawaken the belief in the healing possibilies of logos.

[6] As Harley puts it, "All practitioners, from university graduates to village wise women, had to provide explanations that satisfied those who consulted them, so that medical writing can profitably be seen as competition for the control of meaning rather than as simply self-advertisement" ("Social Construction" 414–15).

practitioners played out also in the protestant print culture of the 1640s, as puritans and Calvinists in particular advocated medicine's popularization. Challenging popular medicine while championing their own, the learned physicians strove for discursive control in a turf war waged as much in print as in practice, and one increasingly populated with some notably vocal competition that included clerics. With logic and grammar, rhetoric complemented the *trivium* of a Renaissance curriculum familiar also to the university-educated clerics who therefore presented the greatest discursive challenge to medical authority. Speaking from a profession equally fraught, those clergy members who deigned to practise medicine not only shared the physicians' rhetorical training but, as much as the physicians drew on the discourse of religion in objecting to the intrusions of their clerical competition, so the clergy counterargued a divinely ordained injunction to heal body and soul.[7]

Thus enacting "the paradox of distinctiveness and openness" Wear identifies as more broadly characteristic of early modern medicine ("Popularization" 19) the impulse both to resist and to protect makes itself known in the physicians' debate with the clergy. Condemning the parson's intrusion while indulging in some discursive interloping of their own, the physicians prove especially intent on defining their profession over-against the clerical as they confirm the importance of rhetoric to an emerging profession.[8] In particular, the vehemence against the so-called Parson–Physition (Sig. $N2_v$/92) expressed by physician John Cotta and his later counterparts James Hart, James Primrose, and Edward Edwards suggests the urgency of learned medicine's protectionist and professionalizing

[7] The physicians may have invoked religion also to counter "the traditional criticism of physicians as greedy atheists" (5) Christi Sumich identifies. John Henry, however, takes a different view in his discussion of medical theory and its relationship to theology, where he notes that medical writers would conventionally avoid "overt clashes of interest" with the clergy and charges of impiety by following a "pattern of medical writing" that would conventionally "begin with expressions of piety and religious devotion" but would later make "no reference to theological considerations" in the medical discussion proper. Henry is careful also to point out that such "apologetic minimalism" should not be construed as "merely lip-service" meant to disguise "covert irreligious sympathies" (97–98). In physician-authored works addressing medicine's conflict of interest with the clergy, however, the pattern is quite different, and the physicians both draw on and challenge clerical discourse in treatises that move beyond mere *apologia* to engage more fully with the theological.

[8] Henry takes a different view in discussing medical theory and theology, suggesting that because medical writers were often associated with impiety, they "avoided any direct confrontation with theology" and thus any "overt clashes of interest" between laity and divinity (97). Rather than engaging in clashes of interest, Henry suggests, medical writers followed convention in opening "with expressions of piety and religious devotion" that preceded a "naturalistic" discussion that "made no reference to theological considerations." It may be that many followed the "pattern of medical writing" but it is also true, Henry admits, that the discursive expression of "deepest beliefs and real intentions" works in ways that "must always remain inscrutable to the historian" (98).

agenda. Responding to a threat explicit not only in the competence of one so obviously accomplished as quondam Professor of Rhetoric turned Anglican priest George Herbert, learned medicine's objections to its clerical rivals rise to the challenge implied by every rhetor capable of analyzing, challenging, and appropriating the physicians' self-fashioning discourse and, like Sir Thomas Browne, therefore denying boundaries impossible to uphold in a culture in which *religio* and *medici* were equally bound by rhetoric.

In his 1612 *A Short Discoverie of the Unobserved Dangers of Severall Sorts of Ignorant and Unconsiderate Practisers of Physicke in England*, John Cotta voices objections that would become amplified later in the century. Cotta elsewhere complains bitterly of other sorts of practitioners and opens the chapter titled "Of beneficed Practisers" by acknowledging that "the grand and most common offenders" are the "divers Astrologers" (Sig. $M4_v$/88), but makes clear that it is the interloping clerics who offend him most.[9] Worst in Cotta's estimation are those who defer to divine providence and dismiss medical treatment altogether. Clerics who mistakenly "perswade the sicke that they have no neede of the Physition," Cotta argues, not only fail to act in a patient's best interest but also deem "God a lyar who expresly saith otherwise" by making "themselves wiser then [sic] their Creator" who "hath ordained the Physition for the good of man" (Sig. $E3_r$/29). Given that physicians since antiquity had invoked divine injunction in arguing for the sanctity of their profession, Cotta's claim is far from unusual. What he and his early modern colleagues do not acknowledge, however, is that to insist that the profession of medicine is akin to the clerical in both origin and healing mandate is to draw authority from while imposing definition on the profession of another.[10]

Though not reticent about asserting the cleric's bounds, Cotta will not suffer the "mercenarie use" of the physician–clerics or allow meddlers reciprocally to enforce his own. A discipline whose parameters are not for others to discern, "in these times," Cotta maintains, healing is "an acquired facultie" rightly practised only by "some speciall and

[9] Cotta also published *A True Discovery of the Empericke* in 1617 and *The Triall of Witch-craft* in 1616, for which Cook suggests he may be better known ("Good Advice" 18). A well-known ranter among the physicians, Cotta offers an extreme (but useful) illustration of the terms of their debate with various interloping and apparently fraudulent practitioners.

[10] Summarizing J. Kosa's 1970 essay, "Entrepreneurship and Charisma in the Medical Profession" (*Social Science and Medicine* 4: 25–40), Gordon Horobin explains that Kosa finds a "charismatic character as peculiar to medicine and clergy" in their professed and perceived "mastery over death" but notes that divinity's has faded, while Kosa also "compares medicine with law and accountancy, and finds that neither of these has, in the 'public mind,' the same aura" (92–93).

select sort of men" (Sig. $M4_v$/88). Cotta's critique "especially" addresses "Ecclesiasticall persons, Vicars and Parsons, who now overflow this kingdome with this alienation of their owne proper offices and duties, and usurpation of others, making their holy calling a linsey wolsey, too narrow for their minds, and therefore making themselves roome in others affairs." In aiming to do both, the "Parson–Physition" (Sig. $N2_v$/92) can do neither job well, and those who attempt metaphorically to weave a hybrid and therefore inferior fabric "impose upon themselves a necessary neglect of both by an unnecessary assumption of the one" (Sig. $M3_v$/86). It may be tempting to infer that the early modern cleric has inherited "the gift of healing in the Apostles [that] was the gift of God," Cotta admits, but such arguments no longer obtain. Insisting that his rivals err in their "want of reverence and respect of order and distinction of callings" (Sig. $M3_v$/86), Cotta offers a scriptural counterargument, reminding such interlopers also that "Saint Paul teacheth every man to walke within his owne calling" (Sig. $M4_v$/88).

Seventeenth-century believers were, of course, obligated to read and interpret the Word for themselves, yet Cotta's borrowings have everything to do with professional self-interest and not personal salvation. In a contest where the university-trained clergy may have been most capable of outdoing the physicians at their own game, Cotta borrows the tools of his adversary as he invokes religious discourse while also insisting that "this fluctuation of these men betweene two callings is offensive to God, scandalous unto religion and good men, and injurious to commonweales." Invoking scripture while complaining of arguments amounting to "presumption borrowing from the face of Divinitie" (Sig. N_r/89), Cotta's argument rhetorically enacts medicine's larger "paradox of distinctiveness and openness" (Wear, "Popularization" 19). Typically for the physicians, however, openness goes only one way: Cotta vehemently excludes clerics from his calling, yet proves their discourse indispensible even to the most indignant of medicine's disciplinary hardliners.

Not long after Cotta's treatise appeared, Northampton physician James Hart penned the anti-clerical argument later included in his 1633 *KΛINKH, or the Diet of the Diseased.*[11] In *A Discourse of the lawless intrusion of Parsons & vicars upon the profession of PHYSICKE with the absurditie of*

[11] The manuscript is held in the Bodleian Library under MS. Rawl. D. 146. A second slightly variant copy available in the British Library, which "appears to have been written later" (369–70), is transcribed in full and appended to Harley's essay, "James Hart of Northampton and the Calvinist Critique of Priest–Physicians: An Unpublished Polemic of the Early 1620s."

the same, the author reiterates that "men may not enter into two callings at once," and are prohibited for three reasons:

> First is God hath disjoined these callings by his word and commandements. Secondly is the practise of the one, hinder the practise of the other. Thirdly is the combining of them together hinder the common good. On these grounds our saviour Christ being the Doctor of the Church, refused to bee judge of inheritance betwixt the two bretheren. And here upon the Apostles begin to doe the office of their owne callings, refused to performe the office of Deacons. (1v)

In his later published treatise, Hart reiterates his complaints about over-reaching parsons, with their small Latin from the grammar schools, who dare to dabble in physic when they would be more properly concerned with their parishioners' souls (12). Hart's book likewise professes to make a case against parson practitioners "they cannot justly except against," maintaining that they should "be ashamed to plead any more this thred-bare excuse of doing good to their neighbours" and, like Cotta, arguing that they would do better to "wait on their Ecclesiasticall functions" (13–15).

Throughout his lengthy argument against clerical intruders, Hart suggests motives other than professional self-interest, indicating that it may have been, as Harley proposes, "the conflict of medical activities with parochial responsibilities that particularly enraged the opponents of the priest–physicians" ("Calvinist Critique" 369).[12] Accordingly, Hart insists that the physician–clerics, "by dividing themselves into two professions," effectively "defraud both of their due attendance" (*Diet* 12). Yet his two-pronged critique had evidently fallen on deaf ears. As Hart goes on to explain, "although this injury hath heretofore, both out of the pulpit, and by the pen of the learned been spoken against; and my selfe also gave a touch thereof in the preface to my former Tractat; yet hath all this as yet produced no reformation" (*Diet* 13). Blaming the recalcitrant offenders for not effecting their necessary reformation, Hart's catalog of arguments made against the physician–clerics recognizes the merits of those made by others, but he also implies that only a "touch" from him is at least as significant as the many speeches and treatises that have come from the pulpit and other learned pens. Including his mere "touch" among what are presumably fully developed arguments, Hart implies that his is nevertheless the most significant. Escalating in force from pulpit to pen to preface

[12] Harley does, however, also acknowledge that the physicians' critiques included "elements of intellectual and economic protectionism" ("Calvinist Critique" 369), a qualification difficult to dispute and characteristic of an argument that aims also to circumscribe the boundaries of another's profession.

over a series of clauses, Hart's amplifying *auxesis* progresses from the transience of oral speech, to the more enduring written, and finally to the permanence of the printed word. Amplified in size as well as significance, the last item in Hart's list, "in the preface to my former Tractat," is also the wordiest, granting by increase the most weight to a prefatory argument assuming climactic place after the lesser "by the pen of the learned" and the least substantial "out of the pulpit."

Those who orate from the pulpit may represent a legitimate profession, but Hart makes clear that it is not equal to his own. Tracing a disciplinary hierarchy in his survey of divinity, law, and medicine, Hart begins with the training of "the able and learned Divine" he distinguishes from "a duns, a droane, or Empiricke divine."[13] Hart's able and learned cleric is instead "trained up in the common schooles of good learning both grammaticall and Philosophicall, and hath, according to standing and seniority, taken such degrees in the Vniversity, as have been by our forefathers thought fit, to grace and adorne learning, and encourage schollers to the pursuite of some eminent excellency in the same." Such learned clerics will then "attaine to some place of the Church, some of greater, and some of lesser value," and those who do particularly well can "againe rise to higher preferment, according to worth, meanes, friends and favour." Diligent from the *trivium*-centred grammar school to preferment, "the worthy, honest, carefull and conscionable Divines (for of such I speake) are laborious and painefull in their callings," and continue to be so, "preaching in season and out of season; administering the Sacraments, and visiting the sicke, &c." Yet Hart takes with one hand what he gives with the other, going on to admit that the industry and effort of the "most laborious" among the clergy can "parallell the Physitians paines," but qualifying his generosity in noting the yet "many other idle ones" not worthy of attention, "there being no need of any comparison with such persons" (*Diet* 19).[14]

Turning to the professions more broadly, Hart begins his discussion "concerning the Physitian" comparing medical education with that of divinity and law. Observing that learned medicine follows the same preparatory curriculum, and "is not behind either of the other two in

[13] The physicians' debate with the so-called empirics (whom Hart implies include some members of the clergy) and other practitioners of practical medicine is taken up in Chapter 2.

[14] Hart goes on to describe legal education, noting that "the Lawyer is likewise trained up in the schooles of good learning, both grammaticall, and sometimes Philosophicall (at least most part of them have spent some time at the Vniversity) and what time is wanting there, it is againe supplied by continuance and studying in some Innes of Court: and after a convenient time they are admitted to the barre to practise their profession" (*Diet* 19).

the ordinary time of his study, and that both in the ordinary grammar-schooles, and the Vniversity," Hart first assumes a posture more defensive than explanatory, but one difficult to take at face value, given that he also offers the marginal reminder that "Physitians study of a far larger extent then [sic] either of the Divine or Lawyer."[15] Quickly turning offensive "concerning the nature and quality of the particular study of this profession," Hart goes on to champion an education not outdone by divinity or law, but one that "is as hard and intricate (if not more) as any of the former two." Hart thus asserts the greater rigors of medical education in an incremental way, opening generously with the negative definition of studies that are "not behind" that quickly become the comparatively "as hard and intricate" and soon surpass in being "(if not more)" so than that of the others. That Hart's parentheses function more emphatically than complementarily becomes clear as he reiterates the distinction with the *epimonic* reminder that the physicians' training is also "of a farre larger extent" (*Diet* 19).[16]

Now surpassing both divinity and law in depth and breadth, learned medicine is defined by a "Theory of Physicke" that is "a great and large field of knowledge" represented by "Authors many and various, and of severall sorts, the Authors of severall nations, and written in severall ages and at severall times: Greeke, Latine, Arabian, and divers others, both antient and modern." Of all these, "the learned Physitian" alone "maketh use."[17] Hart does not doubt that "the Physitian doth yet herein

[15] Referring specifically to sixteenth-century physicians, Pelling and Webster note that "the educated classes of medical practitioner amassed academic qualifications with the same avidity as their twentieth-century counterparts," undergoing training "often so involved and prolonged that by comparison moderns seem distinctly underqualified" (189).

[16] Invoking the London physicians' attempts "to control the many and diverse medical practitioners through the College of Physicians," Cook acknowledges the extent to which the physicians relied on their university education (which invariably included the study of rhetoric), observing that their arguments "had power not just to persuade but to punish" ("Good Advice" 5–6).

[17] Eliot Freidson suggests that "it may be argued that medicine is inappropriately placed in the same category as law and religion because law is man-made and therefore varies from one society to another and religion is based on supernatural revelation which is not amenable to the usual scientific methods of verification, whereas medicine addresses itself to an unchanging biological reality that is as independent of man as the realities of physic and chemistry. The 'laws' of medicine are therefore invariant unlike those of law, and they are empirically verifiable unlike those of religion." Yet Freidson goes on to suggest that "such an argument, however, fails to distinguish physical from social reality," and he therefore insists that "like law and religion, the profession of medicine uses normative criteria to pick out what it is interested in, and that its work constitutes a social reality that is distinct from (and on occasion virtually independent of) physical reality" (206). While Freidson also notes that "medicine is a moral enterprise like law and religion, seeking to uncover and control things that it considers undesirable," it "is kept apart from religion and law because, unlike them, it is believed to rest on an objective scientific foundation that eschews moral evaluation."

goe beyond" divinity and law also "in that hee is, besides his ordinary Theory, to bee acquainted with the whole structure and frame of the body of man, as being the subject whereabout he is conversant." Commanding the abstract and concrete, the learned physician is alone equipped to "considereth exactly the aire, with the alterations thereof" while he "neglecteth not the other Elements, with all the creatures conteined therein, either for the use of food or Physicke." Ending his survey of callings legal, divine, and medical with the telling rhetorical question "what profession can compare with the Physitians paines?" Hart poses an *erotema*, the question to which "none" is the expected answer, that comes with the assurance that the "Physitians practicall imployment" (*Diet* 19) encompasses more than the abstract and theoretical.

Particularly incensed about those interloping clerics who are also suspect "*Romanists,*" and thus pretend to law as well as medicine, Hart insists they are hypocrites to the core. Akin to "*the Divell, that old enemy of our salvation*," who deceives by "*oftentimes transforming himselfe into an Angell of light*," the intruding Romanist meddles in medicine "under colour and pretence of helping the infirmities of their distressed brethren, and of better performing their spirituall functions." The temptation to engage in that which they are not trained "doth draw out of their cloisters, certaine religious persons to read lectures of law, and to administer physicall drugges to the diseased." In Hart's view, such religious persons have no more business tampering in law than medicine. To prevent that "such as are set apart for spirituall imploiment" should "under colour of attaining unto knowledge" see fit to "be intangled with worldly businesse," Hart speaks on behalf of learned medicine in asserting the need for professional exclusion, declaring that "we appoint and ordaine, that it be not permitted to any, after their entrance in religion, and profession of the same in any religious place, to goe abroad againe to heare physicke or law-lectures" (*Diet* 15). Insisting that those who cannot count themselves members of a particular profession be denied any access to its discourse, Hart reveals more than the merely secondary interest in "intellectual and economic protectionism" Harley implies ("Calvinist Critique" 369). For Hart as much as Cotta, defining and protecting the bounds of learned medicine are his primary aim.

Though Freidson articulates a modern scientific view of medicine in which "illness is thought to involve viruses and molecules and thus to constitute a physical reality independent of time, space and changeable moral evaluation" (208), there is little question that early modern medicine sought also to distinguish itself apart from – and above – divinity and law, and that it did so by laying claim to an equally differentiated epistemology.

Baldly expressed in Hart's forbidding of the clerical other even to hear medical lectures is the physicians' aim to fashion a profession of unquestioned distinction.[18] Hart does so by upholding a profession requiring greater "paines" than any other, while Cotta's learned physician takes shape in contrast with the mercenary clergy he opposes. Hart's and Cotta's arguments thus rely on the ethos that is the self-fashioned speaker of Aristotle's trinity of *entechnic* or "artificial" proofs (1356a). The primacy of ethos that, like the complementary proofs of logos and pathos, works by "showing or seeming to show something" (1356a) is made clear also in James Primrose's *Popular Errours: or, the Errours of the People in Physick*, first published in Latin in 1638 and later in Robert Witty's 1651 English translation. The book's fourth chapter, "Of Ministers that Practice Physick," focuses especially on the avarice of the physician–clerics, with Primrose arguing that among them "are many that do seriously, and greedily, and with much gain to themselves, undertake the cure not of souls only, but of bodies likewise, and strive to their utmost to get patients to themselves for the healing of their bodily diseases."[19] Like Cotta, Primrose is intent on fashioning a professional ethos that stands in distinct contrast with the interloping other, but their protectionist desires may be nowhere more evident than in Primrose's attack on the economic motivation that compels divines to intrude "even in such places where there is store of Physicians" (10).

Laying bare the faults of the physician–clerics in the appeal to reason that is the *entechnic* proof of logos, Primrose goes on to tackle, one by one, the points put forth by the clergy in championing their right and ability to practise medicine. Primrose's success in doing so is expressed in one of the book's many paratexts, where one "Doctor Zacutus" lauds the *Popular Errours* as the product of a "learned Author" whose ethos gains much of its persuasive force through a logos that "reasons strongly, answers objections acutely, and refutes wittily" (Sig. B_v).[20] Primrose's careful counterargument

[18] The conflict of physicians and clerics was not exclusive to England. In the 1623 English translation of *The Arraignment of Urines*, Dutch physician Pieter van Foreest (aka Peter Forrest) takes on "*the manifold errors and abuses of ignorant Urine-monging Empirikes, cozening Quacksalvers, women-physitians, and the like stuffe*." If it were "lawfull for every man to meddle with another mans profession," he argues, "then might the Lawyer become a Physitian, the Physitian a Divine, and the Divine all three" and insists that "these mens negligence endangereth the soules of their flockes, while they care most for their fleeces" ("Epistle to the Reader" n. pag.).

[19] It bears noting here that "Galenic medicine," as Wear points out, was also frequently "attacked because of the greed of its practitioners" ("Popularization" 30).

[20] That physicians were as interested in the power of language is certainly suggested, anecdotally at least, by the 1654 publication by professed "Doctor of Physick" John Bulloker of *An English Expositor: Teaching the Interpretation of the hardest words used in our Language* with "sundry Explications, Descriptions, and Discourses." The physician's interest in the specifics of language

is also a response in kind, necessitated by the physician–clerics who also offer up quantities of *atechnic* proof, that is, Aristotle's "inartifical" kind that, unlike the *entechnic* proofs "prepared by method and by 'us,'" are readily available and "not provided by" the rhetor (1355a). In the cleric's case, that proof comes overwhelmingly in scriptural references serving as the *exempla* that illustrate the point. Drawing also on a scriptural arsenal of inartificial proofs while artfully anticipating objections and reasoning strongly, Primrose's logos is in part shaped by the rhetoric of those he disputes.

Of course, early modern writers of all kinds rely on the ready-made evidence of divinity, and their numbers include rhetoricians like Henry Peacham, whose 1593 *Garden of Eloquence* indicates on the title page that its proffered *exempla* are derived "chieflie out of the holie Scriptures."[21] Few, however, go to the lengths of clergyman Lionell Gatford. A professed "Bachelor in Divinity–Physick," Gatford quotes 2 Chronicles 16.12 on the title page of his *Logos Alexipharmakos* – "in his disease he sought not to the Lord, but to the Physitians" – and notes that his directions for dealing with the plague are "*Collected out of the Sole authentick Dispensatory of the chief Physitian both of Soule and Body.*" That the author's method is rooted firmly in his rhetorical education is confirmed by the subtitle describing the book's content as *"certain Aphorismes, premised, and conclusions from them deduced, concerning the Plague, necessary to be known and observed of all, that would either prevent it, or get it cured."* Gatford's explicit mention of aphorisms (in this case scriptural) reminds his reader that his training was not unlike that of the physicians who, in the humanist's *trivium*-centred curriculum, were required to learn scores of the Hippocratic kind. Gatford outdoes those who might be tempted to dispute him, however: taking rhetorical amplification to the extreme, the pages of his text cite biblical references by the dozens, and one page offers up nearly a hundred (13).[22]

Primrose thus seems bound to orchestrate his rebuttal using the tools of his clerical opponents. He does, however, make a point of expressing ambivalence about doing so with the simultaneous insistence that "Diseases are not cured with Eloquence" (3), a snipe that seems aimed

use extended beyond professional or professionalizing interests: Bulloker's is not by any means a specialist lexicon – the first word in his dictionary is *abandon*, and the last is *zone*.

[21] First published posthumously in 1577, Peacham's rhetorical handbook remained popular well into the seventeenth century.

[22] Henry notes that if a recognized "mind–body interdependence created problems for theologians, so did the reformist tradition of founding all one's beliefs on the clear word of scripture" (95); Gatford's parenthetical excesses may thus have done his argument more harm than good.

at an orating clergy.[23] But the physicians' criticisms and their attempts to distance themselves from their clerical rivals belie their own reliance on the evidence of scripture. Hart, in fact, challenges the very foundations of the clerical mandate by pointing not to evidence but to its absence. "I read in the old Testament," he writes, that "*Priests* and *Levites* were commanded to wait and attend upon the service of the Tabernacle first, and afterwards of the Temple," thus invoking scripture to confirm the clerics' religious mandate first to serve God. His scrutiny, however, turned up nothing in the physician–clerics' favour, for "concerning the practice of Physicke," he has found "not one word," thus pointing to a lack of evidentiary support to refute their claim. Hart also uses as much scripture as he can find, making it clear that much of his proof is "taken out of the oracles and aphorismes of the old and new Testament," with secondary support coming from "the antient councells and constitutions of the canon-law," and only "a word or two out of the municipal laws and constitutions of this kingdome" (*Diet* 13). Like Gatford, Hart offers up an abundance of scriptural evidence with marginal references but, unlike Gatford, he does so to conclude that one must "carefully keep within the compasse of his calling, and not rashly rush upon another mans profession" (*Diet* 14). The logos of scripture thus works to buttress the authority of the self-fashioning appeal that is ethos, while a sympathetic pathos appeals to the like-mindedness of an audience familiar with much, most, or all of it. Ultimately, however, logos and pathos serve the dominant appeal of ethos, as rhetoric's artificial proofs work to fashion a speaker whose merits stand in contrast with the doubly flawed physician–cleric, who not only is ill equipped to practise medicine, but cannot even read scripture well.

Even those who sought to reconcile often-competing branches of medicine saw little advantage in rapprochement with the physician–clerics on whose persuasive means they simultaneously relied. Bringing together the

[23] Primrose expresses an ambivalence shared by continental physicians in what Nancy Siraisi describes as rhetoric's "ambiguous reputation." Articulated by writers who "warned physicians against use of persuasion or repeated some version of the truism that patients are cured not by eloquence but by medicine," the ambiguity (or ambivalence) of learned medicine's mistrust of rhetoric is apparent in its ongoing reliance on the epideictic oratory regularly "pronounced at university ceremonies" ("Oratory and Rhetoric" 191). I would add to Siraisi's thesis that treatises like Primrose's very much rely on the *epideictic* in professionalizing arguments that may not be explicitly ceremonial but equally exemplify the rhetoric of praise and blame, a discourse that prompted even Petrarch in his *Invectives against the Doctor* to point out what Nancy Struever identifies as "a glaring disjunction between the doctors' wordy pretentions to know and the difficult nature of the evidence before them" (662). Tellingly, Streuver even describes Petrarch's *Invectives* as "an archetypical Renaissance confrontation of rhetoric and medicine, as well as a primitive encounter of Humanism and science" (659).

theoretical orientation of learned medicine with the hands-on practice of the surgeon, Edward Edwards, a self-proclaimed "Doctor in Physicke," professes in his 1636 *The Analysis of Chyrurgery* to encompass the "Theorique and Practique part thereof."[24] Offering the subtitular notice that the book was "composed for the benefit of all those who desire the knowledge of this worthy Profession," Edwards anticipates the broader audience he addresses in "To the Reader," where he entices with the heavily alliterative and rather florid promise that "I doe not write to fill thy fancies with fables or fruitless lines to fill papers, but I present unto thee a fruitfull garden full of comfortable flowers" (*Analysis* Sig. B_r). In an unabashed display of rhetorical ebullience, Edwards offers a stylistically over-the-top but unmistakable reference to a trope harkening to antiquity and famously expanded in Peacham's *Garden of Eloquence*, a popular guidebook of another kind, that may not ideally represent the decorum an effective *elocutio* demands. What may not meet the fitting standards of rhetoric's third canon, however, may work very well in effecting a pathos aiming to attract "all those who desire the knowledge" the book deigns to impart. Edwards's inclusive aim is further apparent in a volume whose specialized substance is made readily accessible in organized columns accompanied by correlating parentheses clearly pointing to relevant additional information.[25] If accessibility and broad appeal are his primary concerns, then the sometimes-overblown style but carefully wrought arrangement of Edwards's treatise may very well hit the mark. Both verbally and visually, Edwards's treatise seems moved more by a desire for openness than distinction, working not to keep the unlearned out but to fulfill the author's expressed intent of providing benefit to anyone who desires to share the knowledge of his "worthy" and in his case dual "Profession."

To the same end, Edwards extends the correspondence of religion and medicine from the principle of Christian duty to practical application. Edwards's union of medical and spiritual obligation is, of course, far from original or unusual. Even the ancients linked medicine with divinity, and the early moderns maintained with Galen that the art of healing is "the first knowledge or science of humane and divine things" (*Method of Physic*

[24] Even "Galenic medicine," Wear notes, "was self-consciously based on a mixture of experience and book learning," but "it was difficult for the learned physicians to base their claims to a monopoly of expertise upon experience alone, for that pointed in the direction of the empirics and quacks" who were the "hated enemies" ("Popularization" 20) discussed here in Chapter 2.

[25] "The method of tables," notes Stefania Fortuna, "was used in many medical texts in the sixteenth and in the seventeenth century, and the propagator, if not the inventor, is considered to be Pierre de la Ramée" (315), the Petrus Ramus also known for his 1651 *A Compendium of the Art of Logic and Rhetorick*.

Sig. A_r-A_v/1–2) as they invoked a wealth of scriptural evidence to prove the medical calling divine. Accordingly, Edwards argues that the physician functions as an intermediary between God and humanity, taking up the role of divine emissary in "shewing his great goodnesse towards us, by comforting and curing the sore, sicke, and diseased people" (*Analysis* 25). Discernible in a ubiquitous display of God's "great goodness," the language of the divine is also the signature of all things accessible through what the anti-Galenic chemical physician Paracelsus called the "great Volume of the Book of Nature" (66). Of course, the more staunchly Galenic also believed, with Edwards, that anyone fit to practise the "worthy art of medicine" must be "ever serving of God, love and pray unto him daily for his grace and assistance, and consider the end wherefore thou art called to use this worthy faculty" (*Analysis* 25), but Edwards seems here deliberately to inflect the humoral theory and therefore Galenic orientation that shape his analysis proper.[26] Bridging medical epistemologies and practices often in competition, Edwards's words also link physic and surgery with the cleric's divinely mandated duty to serve, extending his rhetorical domain to encompass religion as well as the rival branches of medicine to which he lays equal claim.

In his later 1638 treatise, *The Cure of All Sorts of Fevers*, Edwards nevertheless admits that even from his dual profession is "Divine precept excepted" (Sig. $A2_r$). Professing God's will, he suggests, is out of the physician–surgeon's mandate and, one might surmise, is a role only rightfully claimed by a separate, distinct, and presumably more elevated profession. Yet Edwards also transgresses the very boundaries he affirms as he goes on to articulate "Divine precept" in later reminding his reader that "I need not to relate Scripture saith, God hideth things from the wise and prudent, & openeth them to babes & sucklings."

[26] Edwards's words confirm that seventeenth-century religion and medicine interacted in complex and inconsistent ways. Though the "The links between Protestantism and Paracelsus," Furdell notes, were always clear in a challenge to the medical establishment long compared with Martin Luther's bold confrontation with Roman Catholicism (6), protestants of various persuasions were equally likely to be proponents of Galenism, or practise and uphold a combination of both. Nevertheless, the similarities between the challenges to medical and religious orthodoxy include Paracelsus's writing in German (versus Latin) and his "monumental ego" (6); the iconoclastic physician is also infamous for staging a dramatic burning of medical books. Paracelsus's approach to medicine also grew from both native and classical traditions; as Furdell explains, his work "built a bridge between magic and science" and was predicated on "the Neoplatonic cosmology" (8). Some well-documented epistemological and denominational allegiances attest to the Galenic physicians' tendency to support the episcopacy and their Paracelsian rivals to commit to various religious sects, but there is no fast rule when it comes to early modern allegiances of medicine or religion, with some physicians taking up the tenets of both approaches, while some Galenic physicians, like Hart, were avowed Calvinists though some Paracelsians were not.

Voicing that which he maintains need not be said, Edwards's scriptural invocation marks a paradoxical instance of *paraleptic humilitas* as he goes on to relate what he claims he will not and defers insight to "babes and sucklings." That Edwards immediately follows this patently ironic reminder with the assertion "I accuse none" (*Fevers* Sig. A4_r) heightens the contradictory tendencies of an argument willing also to overlook its earlier, highly accusatory rant against a "rabble of idle droans" made up of the "overwhelming make'shifts" and "smoothing sycophants" whose false professions of physic and surgery are "fit to be unmasked" (*Fevers* Sig. A2_v). Decrying alternative practitioners while claiming to accuse no one, Edwards's simultaneous blame and denial is typical of the sort of contradictions that are a salient feature of a rhetoric that shaped as it gave voice to the wide-ranging debate over who commanded the right and authority to profess medicine. Even as Edwards advocates in his earlier work the "foure speciall things to be considered of every man that will practise this famous worthy art of medicine" and emphasizes that the worthy will do so "not only for thine own gain, as too many doe now abuse it" (*Analysis* 25), he is not averse to invoking scripture in the service of professionalist interests. Like that of his predecessors and colleagues, Edwards's self-fashioning discourse denies the very boundaries it also insists upon.[27]

In a context in which the physicians' "clerical brethren" were equally wont to object "to the knowledge claims of their rivals," Harold Cook points out, the learned clergy were inclined also to make arguments against the physician–clerics, their substance not so different from those the physicians made "against medical empirics."[28] Hence, Cook explains, the clergy

[27] Edwards does acknowledge "that few professions are free of such wretches" as the "dissembling hypocrites" he complains about (*Analysis* Sig. B_r), but his argument may be exceptional in not taking on the clergy directly. Edwards's failure to do so, however, likely has much to do with the context in which he practised medicine. That the clerical rivals who are so often the physician's locus of complaint are conspicuously absent from Edwards's works may suggest that he did not see them as presenting a serious threat to the "learned physician" (*Analysis* Sig. B2_r/3) or, perhaps, that he was unworried by the fact that many of them did choose to practise medicine – a supposition that might in part be explained by the broad applicability of a university education and a curriculum shared in large measure by a clergy who could therefore not be construed as lay. The difference may also be generational, given that Edwards's successors were more intent on denying to the episcopacy-licensed clerics the medical-professional legitimacy the College of Physicians became increasingly intent on claiming for itself. Though *The Analysis of Chyrurgery* was published in 1636, the author tells us that he was aged "81 and six moneths" (Sig. A3_v) at that date. Born around 1555, then, Edwards began practising medicine decades before the century turned, and long before the physicians' dispute with the clerics reached its apex in the 1640s.

[28] As Beier explains, "The term 'empiric' was a general one, intended by the enemies of unauthorised healers to have the same meaning as the word 'quack' has in modern parlance." Some of those practitioners "were in general practice," while others "specialised in the treatment of particular disorders,"

likewise emphasized "the difference between good and bad judgment" and upheld the good version as characteristic of one "whose work was by definition that of 'professing' a view" that entailed "explaining the world so as to keep their listeners within its right order" ("Empiricism" 13). Some clerics were thus as intent as the physicians on keeping proper order, and would also object to the intrusions Cotta, Hart, Primrose, and Edwards also complain about. Perhaps unsurprisingly, those of the episcopacy seemed most likely to lament the medical practice of subordinates who overstepped the bounds of a profession mandated to treat the soul. But, as with the medical-clerical controversy more generally, positions on the debate specific to one denomination or another are difficult to ascribe.

Like future Archbishops of Canterbury and York, Edmund Grindal and Tobie Matthew, some high-ranking clergy were "outraged" and "appalled" at any intermingling of the two professions (Harley, "Calvinist Critique" 363), but erstwhile bishop John Abernethy explicitly brought them together. Insisting on the interdependence of spiritual and physical health in the 1630 second edition of *A Christian and Heavenly Treatise: Containing Physicke for the Soule*, Abernethy makes a forceful appeal to the persuasion of reasoned argument when he writes that "the diseased in body are herein taught, first to seeke health for the soule, that they may the more speedily get health for their body: for God layeth diseases on the body, to restraine, or to punish the diseases of the soule, or to force us to seek spirituall remedies for the same." Taking on the medical practitioner also in invoking 2 Chronicles 16.12 in a reference that follows, Abernethy avers, "We must not be like King Asa, who in his corporall sicknesse sought not his spirituall health in God, but sought to the Physician" (Sig. $A4_r$). For Abernethy as much as Gatford, the art of physical healing is not an entity unto itself, as the physicians would have it, but cannot proceed without the spiritual health advocated by and enacted through the divine Word that is scripture.[29]

and their approaches "differed widely." In any case, "their methods are most often described by enemies" who were "eager to discredit them" (21). The empirics presented a genuine threat to those who opposed them, however, for "there is no doubt that unlearned unlicensed healers were widely consulted" and charged fees "lower than those of licensed surgeons and apothecaries" (27).

[29] Abernethy evidently had some intraprofessional competition as well, notably in the 1616 work of Thomas Adams *Diseases of the Soule: A Discourse Diuine, Morall, and Physicall.* "I haue reason to feare," Adams writes, "that this will be thought but the spawne of that: or an Epitome: or at best, that it is begot out of imitation." Defending the originality of his contribution to the debate, Adams goes on to insist, "Herein I must seriously propose, and engage my credite to the truth thereof: that this was committed to the Stationers hands, perused and allowed by authoritie: yea, and with full time to haue bene printed, and perhaps an impression sold, before that of Master Iohn Abrenethys came out. What dilemma's were in the Book-sellers head, or what reasons for such slacknesse and

As might be expected, clergyman George Herbert argued more plainly in *The Country Parson* on behalf of the right and ability of his profession to practise physical along with spiritual healing.[30] Like that of the physicians, Herbert's professional self-fashioning may have been in large measure motivated by the "pressing and vital issue" Neal Enssle describes as "justifying the Puritan minister's existence in society and his role as spiritual leader," an *exigence* perhaps as pressing to every English clergyman in a context of "rapidly changing political doctrine, economic instability, royal reforms, rising educational standards, and constantly shifting lay expectations of clerical duty and function" (3–4).[31] It may also be that Herbert was further motivated by a shift that saw physicians "called to sickbeds more frequently and earlier than ever before," thereby displacing the clergyman who was once, notes Christi Sumich, "first on the list." In the midst of religion's renewed effort "to govern all aspects and stages of life," Sumich explains, Herbert may have aimed also to bring "death, and even illness, more fully into the scope of religion" (56). Depicting an ideal parson whose role is as all-encompassing as it is indispensable, Herbert's discussion of "The Parson's Completeness" thus opens with the insistence that "the country parson desires to be all to his parish, and not only a pastor, but a lawyer also and a physician" (234). For Herbert, tending to illness as well as death is not mere prerogative but clerical obligation, and his expectation that the parson's duties encompass not two professions but three says as much about his estimation of the cleric's ability as his absolute necessity.[32]

reseruation, are to mee as mysticall, as his profession." Confessing to understand nothing of the bookseller's occupation, Adams nevertheless goes on to write about medical treatment and thereby challenge the physician's authority ("To the Reader" n. pag.).

30 Herbert is, of course, well known as a poet of the plain style, a mode suited to the privileging of profession over class that is a hallmark of *The Country Parson*'s self-fashioning. As Cristina Malcolmson puts it, "The search in *The Temple* for a 'plain' language, the uneasiness over 'quaint words and trim invention'" extends to his clerical conduct book, which is likewise "invested in re-deeming Herbert not only from the unregenerate self, but from the 'character of gentility' which had marked his original modes of self-presentation" (264). In an earlier essay, Michael J. Gallagher more directly aligns Herbert's faith with his rhetoric, arguing the influence of Augustine's Christian orator in "Herbert's theory of style" that renders his "a specifically Christian one" with "a plainness that was capable of power" and a verse style representative of Erich Auerbach's *sermo humilis* (509–10).

31 There has been much discussion of Herbert's doctrinal allegiances and whether his thinking more accurately represents mainstream English protestantism, Calvinism, and even puritanism (see Jeanne Clayton Hunter, "George Herbert and Puritan Piety"). Regardless of the doctrinal inflection of Herbert's beliefs, however, there seems little question that he aimed to shape a parson equipped to respond appropriately to the "shifting lay expectations" of his parishoners.

32 Ronald W. Cooley, in particular, has examined the many ways Herbert participates in the contemporary debate among medical practitioners, showing how his work "engages in a complex process of professional-territorial negotiation, competition, and expansion" (68). Cooley's study also considers the profession of law.

Well prepared to master other disciplines the cleric may be, but the preparation needed to practise medicine responsibly and well is in Herbert's opinion relatively straightforward. Working from knowledge readily accessible to the learned, "is it easy," he writes, "for any scholar to attain to such a measure of physic as may be of much use to him both for himself and others." Achieved merely by "seeing one anatomy, reading one book of physic, having one herbal by him" (235), the medical competence of Herbert's parson is acquired through a program of self-study that stands in marked contrast to the depth, breadth, and rigour of medical training upheld by physicians like Hart. Instead of theories derived from classical authority, Herbert recommends the practical texts of sixteenth-century French physician Jean François Fernel.[33] Tellingly, that Fernelius is "the physic author" who can adequately equip the cleric to play physician has much to do with the character of his rhetoric. Because "he writes briefly, neatly and judiciously," Herbert maintains, "especially let his method of physic be diligently perused as being the practical part and of most use" (235).[34] The terms "neatly and judiciously" accrue much credibility to Fernelius and further imply that success with which "any scholar" can fashion himself a physician comes through careful cultivation of an ethos as appropriate and persuasive as Fernel's, one that extends neat and judicious presentation to a "method of physic" whose propensity for practical application is made apparent also in its mode of delivery. What Herbert's endorsement implies, in other words, is not only that judicious and accessible form corresponds with the usefulness and practicality of the content Fernelius presents, but that the two are mutually and reciprocally constitutive.

Herbert's appreciation for a fitting reciprocity of form and content informs the discourse of a conduct manual everywhere preoccupied with

[33] Learned physicians were not entirely resistant to the practical orientation of alternative practioners, and Fernelius was among those who advocated incorporating empiricism into the Galenist epistemology. "By the mid-sixteenth century," Cook explains, "the felt need of physicians to be in control of the details of nature that were commanded by their rivals was so powerful that the eminent Parisian physician, Jean Fernel, told his peers that empirical knowledge of this kind had to be mastered just as much as learned theory" ("Empiricism" 12).

[34] Herbert's endorsement of the sixteenth-century physician implies his simultaneous rejection of the extensive classical education often concomitant with the advantages of birth. In a context where it sometimes seemed as though "rank now appeared to be determined by wealth and external behavior rather than birth" for "those who sought to be 'genteel'," Malcolmson observes, the "rhetorical self-consciousness so important in both *The Courtier* and *The Prince*" (250–51) also served the parson's self-fashioning. Herbert's corresponding endorsement of a neat and judicious discourse thus corresponds with his simultaneous aim "in general to establish value in employment rather than in family or class" (256) through a rhetoric Malcolmson argues was "used for religious purposes to insure that the churchman's authority will be firmly established in the minds of his parishioners" (251).

decorum. The virtue of apt correspondence in presentation and delivery is as important to Herbert's parson as it is to the physician–author whose work he commends and admires. As Herbert's readers have not failed to note, appropriateness is for him the hallmark of the parson's profession, as form and content work reciprocally to fashion an ethos extending beyond the verbal to the visual.[35] Given that "disorders," as he maintains in the "The Parson's Life," are for Herbert readily "manifest" (204) in both language and presentation, the extent of the parson's spiritual health can be discerned through a bodily appearance that sees outward form shaped by inward content and vice versa.[36] As Malcolmson puts it, "the doctrine of vocation allowed Herbert to tie the externals of social performance to an 'authentic' spirituality" (257). Accordingly, Herbert advocates the parson's dressing in "apparel plain, but reverend, and clean, without spots, or dust, or smell, the purity of this mind breaking out and dilating itself even to his body, clothes, and habitation" (204) to signify as well as encourage the optimal health of body and soul. Achieved partly by redressing inward disorder through careful attention to outward form, the manifest *decorum* of body and spirit confirms the overriding importance of ethos to the parson's fashioning of an authority that cannot, as Christopher Hodgkins points out, simply "be put on with the preacher's robes" (234).[37]

[35] Herbert's concern with ethos is apparent also in other writing. Malcolmson notes that, "in 1618, when George Herbert was twenty-five years old, he wrote to his younger brother Henry in Paris and encouraged him to acquire as much Parisian sophistication as possible, 'whether it be in knowledge, or in fashion, or in words.' Clothes, speech and demeanor should testify boldly to one's quality; a backwardness in dress or a loss of composure is unworthy of a gentleman" (245).

[36] In her discussion of Herbert's poetry, Kate Narveson remarks that "the question" for Herbert "is not whether one could show holiness intentionally and sincerely – that was assumed to be the case" (343). Herbert, notes Christopher Hodgkins, subscribed to the "preaching tradition" articulated in "William Perkins's *Arte of Prophecying*," which "sought the clearest and simplest signs for communicating the preacher's inner life to his hearers." As Hodgkins explains, "This tradition assumed that inner reality preceded outward 'show' and militated against pulpit hypocrisy by insisting that words be matched by everyday deeds" (225). For Narveson as well, there is little question of Herbert's understanding of the reciprocity of inward and outward forms. Herbert's "recognition of a potential slippage between inner and outer," she writes, "did not evoke a skeptical dilemma because the assumption was that the self not only could be structured, but needed structuring. The slippage was susceptible to discipline." Referring also to the visual rhetoric rendering virtue manifest, Narveson suggests that "It is within this conceptual framework that Herbert is addressing how to regulate gesture" and recognizes the poet–cleric's preoccupation with "the decorum of a particular situation" (320–21). Earlier, Narveson notes that "protestant theology condemns the inner/outer self-division," but instead "stipulates as a sign of grace the regeneration of the whole person, whereby the inner spirit matches self-presentation." On this point, she notes disagreement with Debora Shuger's posited "contention that that early modern people operated with a sense of two selves, an external 'performative' and an inner 'pneumatic' self," arguing instead that such a reading "misses this key concern for continuity" discernible in Herbert's verse (317).

[37] That form is not only visible in and shaped by person, garment, and house. According to Herbert, family members needed also to cultivate a decorous ethos that bore witness to as it shaped and

For Herbert, the ideal parson's ethos entails an all-encompassing *decorum* that, as Aristotle would have it, uses all the persuasive means available. The self-fashioned ethos Herbert advocates thus corresponds also with that of the ideally persuasive physician who, Cook notes, established and maintained his professional authority in a context where "Good judgment and advice were considered to be attributes of character at least as much as knowledge." Because it was thought that "knowledge alone would not result in good judgment and advice," Cook explains, the logos of the physician's reason worked in tandem with if not in the service of an ethos bearing witness to the "inner discipline and deep consideration" made visible through the externally borne character ("Good Advice" 4) that served the persuasion of pathos. For the parson as well as the physician, the appeal to audience worked in service of the primary, overarching proof of ethos. In "The Parson's Eye," for instance, Herbert warns against eating "offensively to the company" lest the parson appear "scandalous and uncharitable." An appropriate pathos thus serves an ethos untainted by eating "more than his health or employments will bear," thereby precluding the appearance of a less-than-trustworthy "glutton" or "prodigal" (240).[38] Cultivating an appropriate character ever-attentive to audience, the physician's self-fashioning depended on the "good character" of a professional equipped to present himself in every way as "a man of learning," and one "who could exercise good judgment and advice" instead of merely conveying "information about healing." Yet, as Cook also notes, the physician's authority equally depended on "the long university educations that marked physicians from all other medical practitioners" ("Good Advice" 4), and physicians like Hart are more intent on invoking their "long university education" than the evidence of "inner discipline and deep consideration" Herbert demands of the parson.

Like the physicians, Herbert asserts the primacy of an ethos more important than its supporting proofs or logos or of pathos, yet his professional self is more carefully fashioned than it is asserted by either education or experience. Emphasizing not his command of a particular body of knowledge (which, Herbert's recommendations for medical training suggest, can be easily acquired by the right sort of person), Herbert's professional

supported the parson's fitness: "After religion," Herbert writes in "The Parson in his House," the parson teaches his children "that three things make a complete servant, truth and diligence and neatness or cleanliness" (216).

[38] Narveson observes of Herbert's poetry that "Galenic discourses of health inform the morality of consumption"; thus "harmful merges with sinful" so that "Herbert's sense of spiritual health was shaped by his understanding of physical health" (328).

is most clearly defined by discernible character.[39] If the whole of *The Country Parson* is, as Ronald Cooley claims, "an exercise in professional self-fashioning" (55), then Herbert's is one that privileges the professional over the profession.[40] Though his parson is far from diametrically opposed to the character of Cook's optimal physician, the nature of their respective self-fashioning entails a telling distinction significant in Herbert. In focusing on shaping the individual rather than giving discursive form to the collective, Herbert's rhetoric is decidedly unlike that of a Cotta, Hart, or Primrose (or even of other clergy who wrote in defence of their profession's divinely ordained duty to practise medicine). Standing in marked contrast with the demonstrably collective "intellectual and economic protectionism" of the physicians (Harley, "Calvinist Critique" 369), this is a significant and suggestive difference. Even in what Hodgkins describes as *The Country Parson*'s "apparent commitment to the elite status of the pastor's office," that status is confirmed only by "social contract" with the parishioner (234) in a work that is unique, as Malcolmson claims, in expressing decidedly "country" concerns that stand over against the "Court-stile" propounded in most conduct books (265). Unlike many of the elite practitioners of learned medicine, whose own "Court-stile" validates what Hodgkins describes as Herbert's larger concern "with the ways that the human will to power conspires with or is cloaked by specifically religious language" (227), Herbert presents an authority carefully fashioned by the

[39] Malcolmson argues that Herbert in *The Country Parson* writes the genre of the character, which she defines as one "which claimed to teach its audience how to 'read' men in society and how to 'interpret' their actions as signs of their inner dispositions" (247). Though his " 'country' version of this self-fashioning was an attempt to live the plain style, rather than 'Court-stile,' " she points out, "it nevertheless required an art of self-presentation as elaborate as that detailed by the courtesy books of the time." Moreover, Herbert's self-fashioning contrasts with the elitist insistence of the physicians. As Malcolmson states, Herbert's "art of holiness was meant to be authentic to the extent that it held in check a sense of superiority based on family or class, and to the degree that it disrupted the power of the system of status to determine human value" (265).

[40] Perhaps no example attests more clearly to the credibility of a carefully wrought, persuasive ethos than that of Herbert's fellow poet and healer Henry Vaughan, who likely practised medicine for about forty years with no license and no formal training (see Donald R. Dickson, "Henry Vaughan as Country Doctor"). Vaughan also had problems with his own health. As Graham Hartill points out, "The bulk of his poetry was written in a span of only about seven years, during two of which he is known to have suffered a serious illness, possibly psychological" (12). Vaughan was on the Civil War's losing side, so it may come as no surprise that he suffered from depression, "though he wouldn't have called it such. He wrote his poetry, almost all in the space of seven years, as a way of coming to terms and making sense of his life in the light of his faith" (15). As a sometimes seriously ill religious poet who also practised medicine, Vaughan may serve as a paradigmatic example not only of the extent to which rhetoric, religion, and medicine were interconnected but also of the ostensibly competing epistemologies of the latter; as Dickson observes, it is likely that Vaughan "practiced Galenic medicine even though he espoused Paracelsian ideas" ("Medical Annotations" 427).

individual parson and not claimed by over-wrought assertions of professional belonging.

Herbert's focus on the individual instead of the collective so insistently championed by the learned physicians does not, however, also mean that he refrains from asserting a professional hierarchy that privileges his own. Claiming for his parson an incontrovertible place in law as well as medicine and divinity, Herbert does so not by suggesting an equitable union of the three but by subsuming the legal and the medical into the clerical. In a critical reception summarized by Hodgkins as revealing a sometimes "Elitist, aggressive, manipulative, maneuvering" Herbert, *The Country Parson*'s "emphasis on pastoral surveillance and control over the parish" may indeed cast "a worrisome shadow" (224) over a work whose stylistic plainness – and the presumption of a plain-spoken truth assumed to go along with it – may go far in masking the contradictions that include a will to medicine and law as well as the parish. The Herbert who penned *The Country Parson* had not left his classical and oratorical training behind, and the performance of his in some ways singular rhetoric enacts a simultaneous distinctiveness and openness that may be differently inflected but is just as paradoxical.[41] The poet who wrought "The Windows" may issue the "reminder of the proper identity of the priest" as well as the "remembrance that his exalted role is legitimate and need not be a source of self-aggrandizement or presumption" (90), as Bruce A. Johnson claims, but the priest who wrote the conduct book is not free of the kind of professional presumption more tangible but no more crucial to the physicians' arguments. In a text that, as Cooley puts it, "alternately collapses and expands the distinction between matters medical and matters spiritual" (65) throughout, Herbert expands distinction by laying claim to the medical profession while refusing to shape the parson to fit the physician's mold, and collapses it by fashioning the physician to suit the parson's calling. Herbert's clergy-privileging argument is thus akin to those of the physicians at least to the extent that it also "seeks to enlarge and enclose its own professional field," to borrow Cooley's phrasing, even as it "contests acts of professional closure and enclosure by the medical profession" (68). Sharing tendencies of collapse and distinction, expansion and openness, Herbert's rhetoric is both like and distinct from that of the learned physicians;

[41] Herbert elsewhere, Malcolmson argues, "forcefully distinguishes between rhetorical skill and spirituality, the classical orator and the Christian minister, his former life and his present one," but his self-fashioning exercise leaves little question that "he also welds them together, insisting that the spirit of Christianity can flow into language and rhetorical performance" (263–64).

aiming also to distinguish medicine from religion while privileging the latter, the once-professional rhetorician may do so with less potential to offend, but he nevertheless inscribes some reified boundaries of his own as he lays claim to the calling of another.

Also a religious writer, physician Sir Thomas Browne made a well-known contribution to the medical debate when he joined Primrose on the "popular errors" bandwagon set in motion by French physician Laurent Joubert's 1579 *Erreurs populaires et propos vulgaires*. Acknowledging his fellow Englishman's earlier contribution to the genre, Browne's 1646 *Pseudodoxia Epidemica* opens by noting that "Dr. Primrose hath made a learned & full Discourse of vulgar Errors in Physick." Given that "yet have we discussed but two or three thereof," however, Browne proposes to consider those "vulgar Errors" further ("To the Reader" n. pag.). Echoing the complaints of his treatise-writing colleagues, Browne insists that every profession keep within its calling, for "the wisdome of God hath divided the Genius of men according to the different affaires of the world" and "varied their inclinations according to the variety of Actions to be performed therein." Offensive to God and man are those "who consider not" the divine ordering, thereby "rudely rushing upon professions and wayes of life unequall to their natures." To do so, Browne maintains, is to "dishonour not onely themselves and their functions," and to "pervert the harmony of the whole world." In the larger scheme of things, the *scala naturae* that is the Great Chain of Being determines the place for everyone, and Browne believes that everyone should be in his place: "For if the world went on as God hath ordained it, and were every one implyed in points concordant to their Natures; Professions, Arts and Common-wealths would rise up of themselves" (*Pseudodoxia* Sig. $C2_r$-$C2_v$/19–20; book 1, ch. 5). According to Browne, all would be more harmonious, productive, and learned if all obeyed the dictates of their natural, divinely ordained inclinations and respected the bounds of the professions that go with them. Though *Pseudodoxia* does not specifically address the physician–clerics, its author does regularly invoke the evidence of religion to prove a divinely mandated adherence to professional boundaries.

Medicine and religion are, however, more famously brought together in Browne's 1643 *Religio Medici*.[42] In his earlier exploration of what devotion

[42] Robert Burton, the self-styled "philosopher–divine," who commanded extensive medical learning, offers another notable example of religion and medicine's convergence in his copious *Anatomy of Melancholy*. Burton's work warrants more than cursory attention, however, and doing it justice in the context of religion and medicine could easily take up another book, or at least several chapters. The discussion offered here means to be illustrative rather than exhaustive, and the aim of its first

means to this physician, Browne sometimes shows no qualms about championing his profession in claiming a healing capacity for the physician exceeding that of those who treat the soul, for "sooner than divinity" can presume to cure "pride, or avarice in others," he claims, can he "cure the gout or stone in some." Browne may mean "to speak nothing of the sin against the Holy Ghost, whose cure not only, but whose nature is unknown," but he is willing to rebut the claims of clerics who express the contrary belief that spiritual healing is more effectual and important than physical.[43] Laying more forthright claim to the cleric's domain, Browne professes to outdo the clergy in maintaining that he "can cure vices by physic" even "when they remain incurable by divinity," as his infringement on another's calling moves to the literal with the bold declaration that vices "shall obey my pills when they contemn their precepts" (49; part 2, sec. 9).

Typically for the mercurial Browne, however, hyperbole is quickly deflated by understatement, the *litotic*[44] "I boast nothing" that prefaces his subsequent questioning of his profession's very ontology. Going on to issue the "plainly" bald reminder that "death is the cure of all diseases," Browne quickly concludes that we therefore "all labour against our own cure" (*Religio* 49; part 2, sec. 9). Given that his and his colleagues' best efforts work against the ultimate remedy of death, Browne acknowledges that any attempt to prevent one's ultimate demise is, at least in Christian terms, contradictory and self-defeating. Yet the insistence that the physician can cure vices physical and spiritual remains significant. In voicing the syllogism that brings the physician's healing enterprise to a point of utter futility – and his profession to a position of radical uncertainty – Browne works subtly to distinguish medical epistemology from that of divinity. Unlike the clerics who have "to the power of human reason, endeavoured

part is to offer a context for considering the women writers who are the focus of Part II. Issues of economy and focus aside, my interest in Browne over Burton has also to do with fact that the former was a practising physician who wrote about religion, just as Herbert was a practising cleric who advocated for the parson's practice of medicine. But Burton, Angus Gowland notes, had "no pretence of being a practitioner" (98).

43 "We are sensible enough of the least sicknesses of the flesh & of the smallest pin, poynting into the remotest part of the body," Abernethy writes, "but as for spirituall diseases, they are both many, and most easily contracted; hardly eschewed: hardlier found, and felt: and most hardly helped, and healed" (2). Abernethy may claim better to help and to heal than the physician, but he does keep more firmly within his professional compass in focusing primarily on the spiritual.

44 Gideon Burton's *Silva Rhetoricae* defines *litotes* as "Deliberate understatement, especially when expressing a thought by denying its opposite," but also points out that "the Ad Herennium author suggests litotes as a means of expressing modesty (downplaying one's accomplishments) in order to gain the audience's favor." Browne's *litotes* accords with the latter definition (Web. 4 Feb. 2012. <http://rhetoric.byu.edu/>).

to make all go in a literal meaning," he claims comfortably to accept the uncertainty that comes with "a great deal of obscurity" from scripture identified in this instance as "the first chapters of Genesis" (*Religio* 24–25; part I, sec. 34).[45] Browne thus makes an interpretive distinction other treatise-writing physicians miss. More subtle than his colleagues, he willingly embraces uncertainty and values the obscurity he recognizes yet the crude exegete cannot accept in his overriding compulsion to impose interpretive closure on the language that must ever resist it.[46] As aware as Foucault of "an exegesis" ever linked to an "ever secret" and "ever beyond itself" divine Word (Intro.), Browne may invoke the discourse of religion, but does so with the understanding that his argument (let alone his professional labours) may very well resolve nothing. At the same time, his words lend unspoken support to Hart's insistence that the education of the physician does indeed exceed that of the cleric in rigour as well as breadth and depth as he asserts a reasoning capacity borne witness by an interpretive understanding belonging to this physician alone.

Transcending the rhetorical abuse implied by the cleric's text-wrenching literalism, Browne's own discourse figures an ethos more open and uncertain than distinctive and closed. Challenging even the reader's own certainty, Browne dashes expectations in expressing, for instance, the belief "that all that use sorceries, incantations, and spells, are not witches, or, as we term them, magicians." The doubting Browne of *Religio Medici* is far less sure that those who practise such deceptive arts can indeed be easily labelled as one or the other sort of interloper he readily identifies in *Pseudodoxia*. Rather than ranting of witches and necromancers, Browne moves quickly (and surprisingly) to connect magic to rhetoric's *trivial* companion and longstanding rival: "Thus, I think, at first, a great part of philosophy was witchcraft; which," he explains, "being afterward derived to one another, proved but philosophy, and was indeed no more than the honest effects of nature: – what invented by us, is philosophy; learned from him, is magick" (*Religio* 22; part I, sec. 31). Browne thus collapses the distinctions between epistemologies of inherited knowledge and specious

[45] Such literal reading is identified as a problem in *Pseudodoxia Epidemica* as well, where Browne's discussion of deceptive fallacies includes the observation that "by this way many errors crept in and perverted the doctrine of Pythagoras, whilest men received his precepts in a different sense from his intention, converting Metaphors into proprieties, and receiving as litterall expressions, obscure and involved truths" (13; book I, ch. 4).

[46] Ingo Berensmeyer characterizes Browne's thinking about religion, rhetoric, and politics in a way that parallels Browne's thinking about religion and medicine. "The basic condition for his perspective on rhetoric, religion, and politics," Berensmeyer observes, "is epistemological: the uncertainty of knowledge leads the intellectual toward humility, moderation, and skepticism" (126).

magic; both are rooted in "witchcraft" ontologically no different from philosophy to the extent that both are "no more than the honest effects of nature." Though Browne makes clear in *Pseudodoxia* that "the mortallest enemy unto knowledge," is such derived philosophy, which "hath done the greatest execution upon truth, hath beene a peremptory adhesion unto Authority, and more especially the establishing of our beliefe upon the dictates of Antiquities" (20; book 1, ch. 6), his link with witchcraft in *Religio Medici* is suggestive in a way the later work is not. What Browne points to here is the futility of even trying to assert differences between opposing yet equally nebulous epistemologies, ways of knowing whose shared origin belies their oft-professed and largely constructed differences.

Hence the nuanced, tentative, and exploratory mode of *Religio Medici* is very different in both substance and form from the unabashedly professionalizing treatises that include Browne's *Pseudodoxia*. This distinction may, of course, have much to do with the private purpose of the former and the public intent of the latter, the earlier work devised as an outlet for the musings of the religious man and the later penned to serve the interests of his profession.[47] Yet *Religio Medici* produced a response very different from what may well have been private intentions. Ironically and in large measure because of *Religio Medici*, Browne has become as well or better known as a literary figure than the scientific and exegetical thinker he presents to the public in *Pseudodoxia*.[48] The resulting focus on his much-lauded prose style has thus long privileged form over content, to the extent that the ways in which its religious expression is specifically that of a physician has, in a perhaps greater irony, garnered comparatively little attention – and sometimes none.[49] Such an oversight may, of course, have much to

[47] It is well known that Browne was not keen to publish his manuscript, and the implications for the oft-discussed tension of private and public have long been taken up by his readers. It is arguable, however, that religion for Browne "is an intersection between the private and public domains, a place where one side of the distinction seeps into and penetrates the other" (122), a point Berensmeyer makes that parallels my own reading of religion and medicine in Browne.

[48] As recently as 2006, Berensmeyer complained this has been the case "ever since the Romantics discovered him as one of their precursors." Rather than paying attention to his politics, says Berensmeyer, Browne "was read for his 'mere style,' his artful and presumably self-conscious virtuoso use of language," not "for what he might have had to say but rather for the way he phrased it." That Berensmeyer qualifies the "what he might have had to say" with "whatever it was" attests to the complexity and difficulty of Browne's thinking, and thus the tendency of readers either to admire him as "supremely baroque and literary" or condemn him "as self-indulgent and politically ineffective" (113). With Berensmeyer, I would argue "that readings of Browne as a mere stylist are flawed by conceptual and historical misunderstandings" (114) and that rhetoric, religion, and medicine are as politically important as the rhetoric, religion, and politics Berensmeyer sees as "clearly interrelated and intersecting" in *Religio Medici*.

[49] Ronald Huebert points out in his sketch of Browne's seventeenth- to twentieth-century reception history that critics like Michael Wilding who fail even to "acknowledge that Browne was a

do with Browne's interest in *Religio Medici* as a private text written for his own purposes; that the work served as much as a tool for exploring his own thoughts as a means of expressing of them surely goes a long way toward explaining why Browne's *religio* seems not to have a whole lot to do with *medici*.

Yet *Religio Medici* has not gone unnoticed by some medical historians, particularly in relation to those specialties that focus on the mysteries and complexities of the mind.[50] What may represent a rather prescient awareness on Browne's part becomes more apparent in light of recent theories and studies of empathy, "the most rigorous" of which, Rebecca Garden explains, "address empathy as a faculty that involves both feeling and reason" ("Empathy" 552).[51] Browne the subtle reasoner is also the physician of feeling who famously wrote that "I never hear the toll of a passing bell, though in my mirth, without my prayers and best wishes for the departing spirit," and for whom religion and medicine were inseparable, for "I cannot go to cure the body of my patient," he goes on, "but I forget my profession, and call unto God for his soul" (*Religio* 46; part 2, sec. 6). Reading *Religio Medici* from the perspective of empathy, in fact, makes it most clear that the physician who "could never divide myself from any man upon the difference of an opinion, or be angry with his judgment for not agreeing with me in that from which, perhaps, within a few days, I should dissent myself" (5; part 1, sec. 6) sees his faith and the discourse that defined it as

medical doctor" altogether erase "the Medici of the book's title." Huebert's telling "question of omission" (130) may apply to most if not all of Browne's readers. A. Batty Shaw does, however, note that Browne has attracted attention from some historians of medicine, notably Jerome Mortimer Schneck, whose 1960 *History of Psychiatry* offered "an authoritative study of Browne's psychological awareness and intuitiveness" that draws on "many passages from Browne's writings" (42).

50 Shaw explains that Schneck's 1960 *History of Psychiatry* presented "an authoritative study of Browne's psychological awareness and intuitiveness," supported and "illustrated by many passages from Browne's writings." Shaw goes on to note that "Schneck has shown that Browne made a number of perceptive psychological and psychiatric observations that can only now be appreciated in the light of recent trends in medico psychological study" (42). Shaw, however, also points to Browne's limitations as a physician and scientist. "In spite of his great learning and his acute powers of observation," he opines, "it is remarkable that at a time of such revolution in science and knowledge he made no other observation in clinical medicine than to describe adipocere." Even though "he has been called 'a hunter of oddities and strangenesses'," Shaw suspects "that this sometimes clouded his appraisal of a clinical situation." Evidently, Browne was also guilty of being unable to "see through some of the common errors of his age such as the efficacy of the King touching for scrofula or the value of Powder of Sympathy" (42).

51 Shaw notes that Schneck's *History of Psychiatry* "has shown that Browne made a number of perceptive psychological and psychiatric observations that can only now be appreciated in the light of recent trends in medico psychological study" (42). I would add that Browne's unique understanding of empathy is similarly accessible to us in hindsight in light of even more recent studies of empathy in medical practice.

not separate from but very closely allied with that of a profession whose self-fashioning was as slippery and contentious as the religious beliefs that in a mere "few days" might also be met with "dissent." For the Browne of *Religio Medici*, professional epistemology is so inextricably bound up with his beliefs about religion that the two offices require little or no explicit distinction. *Religio Medici* is everywhere marked by the ethos of this particular practitioner, and it is one that is both the product and the expression of a rhetoric inflected to uphold without contradiction a *via media* more open and inclusive than distinctive and exclusionary.

That Browne writes simultaneously as a man of religion and medicine he makes most clear in a metaphor that acknowledges as it bridges their respective ways of knowing: "there are two books from whence I collect my divinity," he writes, "Besides that written one of God, another of his servant, nature, that universal and publick manuscript, that lies expansed unto the eyes of all" (*Religio* 12; part 1, sec. 16). Through the divine Word most visibly manifest in scripture and in the ultimately readable yet obscured signature of all things thought imprinted throughout the physical world, Browne makes clear that he reads as spiritual believer and bodily healer. Seldom, though, do Browne's *religio* and *medici* unite so clearly or readily. Hence critics have long puzzled over the difficulty of accessing Browne's political and professional as well as religious beliefs, and the notion of the complexity, and even indeterminacy, of his *Religio Medici* has been well trod over.[52] Of course, this problem has much to do with his practising of a profession whose theory, as Stephen Pender remarks, "was charged with inconsistency and contradiction," and its "practice with uncertainty and risk" ("Uncertainty" 4). Browne thus evinces an understanding of rhetoric whose nature is wholly consistent with that of his profession, a discipline whose application may be, as Berensmeyer puts it, equally "performative" and "action-oriented" yet provides "a provisional, contingent, or 'collaterall' access to truth that is admittedly imperfect and subject to revision" rather than "a stable epistemology" (115). Recognizing the contradictions (as well as the consistencies) that lie within the tentative *Religio Medici* and between it and the adamant *Pseudodoxia Epidemica* can thus do more to clarify than complicate the oft-iterated problem of how Browne's religious tenets are specifically those of a physician. Despite Browne's prefatory claim in "To the Reader" that "wee are not Magisteriall

[52] Huebert admits that "Browne's habit of piling qualification upon qualification, of offering a number of ways to grasp a single idea, of allowing for changes and instabilities within his own mental geography, can test the patience of any reader" (130).

in opinions, nor have wee Dictator-like obtruded our conceptions" (n. pag.), the *Pseudodoxia* imparts an assuredness contrasting with the radical uncertainty of *Religio Medici*, uniting in a single author a recognition of human achievement that stands over against a more salient understanding of its infinite shortcomings. Taken together, *Pseudodoxia* and *Religio Medici* give voice to what Thomas Greene once styled "two faces of a single coin" (9).[53]

Those conflicting impulses of "humanist pride and humanist despair" (Greene 9) are even more pointedly illustrated in the 1621 treatise *Physicke for Body and Soule: Shewing that the Maladies of the one, proceede from the sinnes of the other*. Not a physician writing of religion but a clergyman writing of physic, "Bachelor of Divinitie" Edward Heron professes to offer "a remedie against both" maladies of body and soul. In doing so, Heron sometimes relies on the evidence of Christ's healing miracles, in one instance offering up an analogy that, by any rhetor's standards, meets the bringing-before-the-eyes criterion Aristotle requires of a memorable and effective *enargeia*. Writing of the "two-fold nette" used by Christ "to catch and drawe men unto him," he dubs the first the "net of wonders." According to Heron, Christ in this first net "caught those many who beleeved in his name, when they saw the miracles which He did," while in the second, which he calls the net of words, "He enclosed his very enemies, those Officers who were sent to apprehend." Those enemies, he says, "were so entangled in the net of his heavenly doctrine, that they had no power to lay violent hands upon him, but returned with this answer" from John 7.46, that "never man spake as that man did" (1–2). Heron goes on to recount how the divine healer also used both nets "in the recovering of a certain poore, lame, and diseased man," explaining that "first He heales him with the bare word of his mouth" and then "He cast upon him the net of his words and doctrine" (2). Heron's metaphor is as suggestive as it is striking, indicating as it does that there is no escaping the wonder or power of the *Logos* incarnate manifest in "the concrete images" of an "ever secret" divine Word that conceals even as it seems to show. Hence Heron's two-fold net of wonder and words bears "the stigmatas of its historical origin" (Foucault, Intro.) in ominous insinuation of stunned and therefore inevitable capture. Though the effects of Christ's net are in theory only good and desirable, Heron's imagery carries the vivid reminder that language may indeed serve opposing purposes at the same time.

[53] Berensmeyer draws a similar analogy in noting that "for Browne, truth is (at the very least) 'double-faced,' and the two faces or facets of truth are not mutually exclusive but 'collaterall' " (126).

The "two faces" of a rhetoric simultaneously open and distinctive may be most readily apparent in early modern medicine's dispute with the physician–clerics. Though one face of the coin aims to exclude the interloping clergy, its flip side invokes the adversary's mode in championing a profession whose most vocal defenders lack Browne's subtlety. Failing to recognize the "epistemology of contingency" (Berensmeyer 126) that also shapes Browne's rhetoric, those less-aware physicians fail to recognize that the necessity they infer from the *exigence* of the moment most often works against the demands of their particular situation; hence the physicians cannot help but fashion a profession that, rhetorically at least, is not so different from that of the clerics they simultaneously and paradoxically insist on opposing. Because the physicians cannot deny their epistemic dependence on language always rooted in the divine Word, they can neither firmly nor consistently uphold the distinction between the spiritual healing assigned to the clerics and the physical healing to which they lay exclusive claim. Despite the physicians' protests to the contrary, what they wish to construe as distinct and incompatible discourse communities, like Browne's philosophy and witchcraft, turn out to be epistemologically as well as rhetorically linked.[54]

In part because of the intersecting nature of discourses medical and religious, Sumich argues, seventeenth-century "physicians were able to present a convincing enough portrayal of themselves as respectable and their services as valuable" even "when there was precious little more than perception to recommend them" (5). By the century's end, however, the physicians were moving away from the earlier dependence on the Word their speculative epistemology had hitherto required. Robert Godfrey illustrates the difference quite clearly in his *Various Injuries & Abuses in Chymical and Galenical Physick* of 1674, where he asserts that "for if Hippocrates and Galen were well-studied and good Linguist: yet 'tis to be understood, that they spent not their whole time about the Nominative case and the Verb, or in Readings only, and subscribing to the errors of their Predecessors." Rather than losing themselves and their acolytes in language – or Browne's famous "mystery" (*Religio* 7; part 1, sec. 9) – medicine's classical fathers,

[54] Long obscured by the certainty of "biological medicine," the shared perspectives of medicine and religion so visible in the seventeenth century have, notes Brian Stock, become apparent "for the first time in centuries." Giving voice to a paradigm once intently focused on a knowable body but increasingly inclusive of an elusive mind and spirit also means that, Stock explains, "a vocabulary once reserved for religion has been transferred to medicine" as "medical perspectives based on mind–body relations" have reciprocally "invaded the field of religion" (490–94) in discourses that represent not a new but a newly awakened rhetoric akin to its early modern counterpart in encompassing discourses of body and soul.

Godfrey argues, devoted more time to *praxis* than theory, spending "the greatest part in Materia Medica, and in procuring such noble Remedies as might credit a Physician, and cure the Diseases of their Age" (7). By Godfrey's day, the rift between the practical and theoretical, the medical and the spiritual, had become clear and ever-widening, the discourse of the learned physicians no longer so dependent on religion to give voice and form to their self-fashioning. By the early decades of the eighteenth century, Furdell points out, "the science and practice of medicine had gradually disengaged from spiritual matters" (92), and, as we shall see, its seventeenth-century antecedent laid growing claim to once-antithetical ways of knowing as, notes Cook, "English society increasingly came to value professional authority based on educated judgment less and to value one based on empirical experience and efficacy more" ("Good Advice" 25).

CHAPTER 2

"Onely the Learned" *Physicians, Empirics, and Women*

Heralded on its title page as "absolutely necessary for directing all Practitioners" and "sufficient thorowly to acquaint any judicious man with all the Principles of *Physick* or *Medicine,*" Peter English's *Galen's Method* responded to growing demand for medical knowledge. Even as his 1656 translation offered medical "Principles" and "Applications" in vernacular form, however, it aimed also to preserve the distinction of a text yet deemed to surpass "all others." Announcing "thy Darling" book's broad accessibility to the "Gentle Reader," English lauds to his "gentle" audience a work "matchless in its kind" and therefore "absolutely necessary for directing thee in any practice of *Physick.*" Asserting that it is "impossible to administer any Cure safely" without consulting the second-century Roman physician, English may be responding directly to Nicholas Culpeper, whose 1652 version of Galen was infamously preceded by his unauthorized 1649 translation of the London College of Physicians' protected pharmacopoeia.[1] Making available what had hitherto been inaccessible to those without Greek or Latin, Culpeper's *A Physicall Directory* accelerated medicine's popularization, Elizabeth Lane

[1] Culpeper "wished to overthrow the physicians," and his staunch defence of liberty was "welcomed by the parliamentary press," Harold Cook notes, and "caused the College much embarrassment" (*Medical Regime* 121). It is telling of Culpeper's influence as well that "three-quarters of the vernacular medical books published between 1641 and 1740 appeared in multiple editions" (Fissell, "Marketplace" 111). Because apothecaries like Culpeper believed that "teaching was a necessary concomitant of healing," explains Louis G. Kelly, "they were prolific translators of medical texts, both standard and non-standard, and they also compiled medical handbooks" (166); the apothecaries were also alchemists who "practised their profession within a complex of religious and political ideas that saw no boundary between religion, physical science, and medicine" (163). Culpeper refused to defer to authority of any kind and "lambasted all kinds of hierarchical authority, monarchical, aristocratic, episcopal or medical" as he "virtually reinvented vernacular medical publishing" (Fissell 118). Wear proposes that Culpeper may have been a Leveller ("Popularization" 31), an interpretation that reinforces and may in part explain his populist desires. Among numerous other works on astrology and medicine, Patrick Curry's *DNB* entry notes, Culpeper went on to publish in 1651 his *Directory for Midwives*, and in 1652 his popular, self-authored reference, *The English Physitian*.

Furdell explains, by intensifying public demand for more in the way of "do-it-yourself prescriptions" (98). English, however, counterargues that any remedy achieved without Galen's guidance succeeds only "at randome" by a method akin to "a blind man throwing his staffe at a dog" (n. pag.) as he insists that neither translated form nor proclaimed usefulness be permitted to compromise the ancient authority on which the physicians predicated their own.[2]

Earlier, the self-identified "Practitioner in Physick" Thomas Sherwood professed to share his medical knowledge in his 1641 *The Charitable Pestmaster, Or, the Cure of the Plague* but, like English, did so only with the caveat that "all the excellent Medicines that are in the Apothecaries Shop" (5) are of little use to those who lack the physicians' learning. For Sherwood as well, remedies are effective only when ministered by the "skilfull Physician," who can do "more with a cup of warme drinke in the cure of the Plague, or any Fever" than "the ignorant" (5) can hope to accomplish even with all of the medical information available. Without the right kind of education, Sherwood argues, the literate but unlearned cannot hope to achieve the healing ability of the physician, whose efficacious "warme drinke" results not from experience but knowledge acquired with little practical training. Even as he sought for his guide the protection of the London College, however, Sherwood also understood that learned medicine's professionalizing enterprise depended as much on popular assent as its own self-fashioning. Though physicians posited their singular education against the practical knowledge they could not exclusively claim, they knew as well as anyone that "there was," as Beier points out, "no consensus in the general population that licensed healers were the sole authorities in medical matters" (5) and, in response, they inflected their knowledge with that of their competition as they made it more readily available by publishing in the vernacular.

[2] As with the many early modern translations that "digested, popularized, and made accessible the classical works of Hippocrates and Galen," English's perhaps "suggests a model of medical knowledge coming down in a diluted form from the top to the reading public." Such a model, Wear elaborates, inscribes a distinction "between medical writer and reader, or between learned source and popular author" that implies "the movement or trickle down of that knowledge from high culture to low" ("Popularization" 19). Though those distinctions may be as blurred as Wear goes on to argue, there remains little question that English upholds some degree of division between author, translator, and reader, and that the latter assumes the lowest place. Thomas Gale's 1566 translation, *Certaine Workes of Galens, called Methodus Medendi*, predated English's by nearly a century and, in aiming "to make everie bodie cunning in the arte of medicine, with setting foorth of these my works in the English tongue," the translator disclaims any intention "to instruct those which be great learned men" ("The Epistle Dedicatorie" n. pag.). Gale's modesty and evident sincerity contrast with English's desire to appease the public while protecting the hierarchy.

Aware of a growing appreciation for the practical knowledge of "naturalists, empirics, mathematicians, and chemical physicians" who, John V. Pickstone notes, "increasingly took the business" (504), the physicians nevertheless complained ad nauseam about the derisively dubbed "empirics," the medical rivals whose numbers often included licensed surgeons and apothecaries, as well as the women who sometimes worked as "petticoat" physicians or surgeons but more often practised healing as an extension of their domestic duties.[3] Thus also seeking to uphold an epistemological divide bound by ways of knowing construed as deeply and irrefutably irreconcilable, learned medicine's challenges to non-clerical rivals proved more intent on championing theory over practise. Defining the physician over against an often-undifferentiated empirical other, asserting the value of the learned physicians' bookish epistemology over the practical understanding of myriad medical rivals, deploying linguistic expertise in the service of learned medicine's intellectual protectionism and self-fashioning, and demonstrating the incapacity of women to achieve the learning or intellectual prowess that distinguished the true physician, the rhetoric of early modern medicine remained intently exclusionary even at its most popularizing.[4] Laying discursive claim to the tenets and principles of an epistemology they had once vocally opposed while upholding their own distinctiveness, the physicians' "protracted advancement towards professionalization" (Churchill 232) was well served by arguments that worked paradoxically but to desired effect. Predicating their anti-quackery arguments on a logos unstable in its many contradictions, however, learned medicine insists but does not reasonably show that the physician is, as Cotta would have it, the only "true artist."[5]

[3] Pelling and Webster describe "the academically educated physician," who spent seven years studying for the MA and a "further seven years or more accumulating medical qualifications," as "a humanistically inclined scholar, familiar alike with classical tongues and the medical science" (189). In practice, as Pickstone describes it, "the main activity of the traditional Galenic physician" was "to interpret lives in terms of 'physiology.' " The physician's heuristic training, he points out, was the marker of "high-status knowledge that made medicine a liberal art rather than a craft," and one articulated with "the language of diagnosis and prognosis and of the rhetorics that combined social and natural meanings." As with "the physical sciences of the seventeenth century" (504), Pickstone implies, medicine responded increasingly to epistemological change as well as the demands of a "medical marketplace" in which, Jenner and Wallace note, "in any year a sick person might visit a wart-charmer, get a remedy from a neighbour or bookseller, pay for a surgeon and hire a horse leech" (2).

[4] Beier notes that the "anti-quack" literature "intended to inform, to shock, to convice and to entertain," and may "resemble nothing more than very early examples of yellow journalism, complete with villains, heroes, victims and the pleas for a public meting out of justice to all concerned" (38). Yet their vitriol surely underscores the importance of rhetoric – however abused and abusive – to the physicians' professionalizing agenda.

[5] "The true Artist his right description and election" is the title of the Third Book of Cotta's *A Short Discoverie*.

Relying on empirical persuasion while stridently championing the Galenic, the learned physicians invoke rival epistemologies in deploying a logos as open to discursive appropriation as it is intent on proving distinction. James Hart, for instance, figures a medical understanding predicated on the signature of all things famously propounded by Paracelsus and others when he argues that the learned physician "searcheth into the secret and abstrusest closet and cabinet of nature, inquiring into the natures and qualities both of simples and compounds in the universall world" (*Diet* 19).[6] Though obscured by what Hart calls nature's "closet and cabinet," the remedies of practical medicine were thought discernible from "the universall world," and could thus be translated into correspondingly curative "simples and compounds." Yet Hart insists on positing a learned physician defined by singular training and ability. Indeed, "within the compasse of his profession," the physician is equipped not only to probe "the secret and abstusest" closet of nature but "all things sublunary." Given that even "the Heavens themselves come within the precincts of his knowledge" (*Diet* 19), Hart's physician commands knowledge so broad and deep that his bona fide professional becomes undefinable. Yet Hart's logos gives shape to an argument more cautious than such bold overreaching may imply. Because the learned physician pursues such vast knowledge "not in that superstitious manner as some doe" but responsibly and credibly, he stands above and apart from the illegitimate medical practices some might erroneously "tye us thereunto" (*Diet* 19). No dilettante, dabbler, or imposter, Hart's learned physician may lay preposterous claim to all knowledge, yet is upheld as insistently distinct from the unlearned and therefore specious interloper.

[6] The differences between learned and practical medicine were intensified by the sixteenth-century work of the continental astrologist, alchemist, and physician Paracelsus, whose growing influence coincided with medicine's popularization. Questioning the norms of learned medicine, Paracelsus's work on chemical therapy interrogated a practice long rooted in Galenic humoral theory, and training that included virtually no hands-on experience. Hence Paracelsian practitioners, who by and large did not include the learned physicians, "denounced Galenists" as the book trade strove to meet the demand "for ever more information, discussion, and advice about sickness and well-being" it helped to create (Furdell 12–28). Though it is true that many of the learned physicians, particularly those who were College members, more usually resisted Parcelsianism in all of its manifestations and inflections, the allegiances of seventeenth-century medicine were no more uniformly epistemologically than doctrinally aligned. Particularly in the mid- to late century, physicians adjusted their thinking and their practice away from the Galenic and toward the Paracelsian, and the epistemological distinctions between and within ways of knowing thought to be incompatible became even less clear. Hart, however, was as opposed to "unlearned medicine" as he was "to unlearned religion" (Harley, "Calvinist Critique" 367) and, as Peter Elmer explains, "a new emphasis upon the Bible as a source of natural wisdom is also evident in the writings of the English Paracelsians, knowledge which was generally believed to complement the evidence gleaned from that other book of God, 'the Book of Nature'" ("Puritan Revolution" 16).

The paradox of Hart's argument becomes especially glaring in light of the learned physicians' objections to those imposters who, as Galen laments in English's translation, made equally pretentious claim to "the whole Art of *Empyricks.*" Discredited through claims as impossibly vast as those of Hart's physician, the empiric's knowledge cannot be genuine, Galen reasons, also because it is founded on "nothing else but some observation and remembrance of those things which appear to have some connexion among themselves" (*Galen's Method* 28). As he asserts a singular ability to make connections among the simples and compounds discerned from nature's darkest cabinet, Hart is thus careful also to make clear that he champions only "the learned Physitian" while parenthetically emphasizing that "(for of such, and not of ignorant and unlearned Empirickes I here speake)" (*Diet* 19). Offering an explanatory aside that does less to amplify his argument than underscore its potential undoing by the contradiction he willfully ignores, Hart takes an opportunistic jab at the rival "unlearned Empirickes." Hart's *paraleptic* assertion draws attention to what he professes not to write of, and what he elsewhere defines as all who "undertaketh the practice of this profession by meanes of some receits, or traditionary medicines," a category that includes the expected "*Women Physitians, Surgeons, ignorant Apothecaries, fugitive Physicians*" as well as "*Mountebankes, Quack-salvers, Ephermeriades-masters,* and many more of this stamp" (2).[7]

Hart may scoff at "receits" and "traditionary medicines," but appeals to the ancient equivalent in commending "punctuall" Hippocrates, the "Father of Physicians," for "prescribing the exact periods and severall circumstances of the diet in acute diseases of his daies" (2). Arguing that the diseases of a particular day demand treatments that the fixed formulæ of "traditionary medicines" cannot take into account, the logos of Hart's reasoning aligns with that of other physicians. Noting Hippocrates's skill with prescriptions and extolling the merits of remedies wrought from nature's secrets, Hart addresses anticipated objections to the privileging of theory over praxis as he also emphasizes the "exact periods and severall circumstances" that render effective treatment context dependent. Yet

[7] Physicians, notes Cook, "self-consciously used the word 'profession' with regard to themselves and to no other medical practitioners," and did so with the aim of "clearly identifying their profession as something other than a mere occupation" ("Good Advice" 4). Freidson observes that "the professional is an expert because he is thought to possess some special knowledge unavailable to laymen who have not gone through his special course of professional training" (338), and there is little question that Hart defines himself and his specialized knowledge over against the "unlearned Empirickes" he opposes.

Hart cannot have it both ways, and intentions do not wholly coincide with effect. Implying that learned medicine may not be utterly divorced in application from the empirics he categorically disdains, Hart's anticipatory *procatalepses* may author his own defeat; at the same time, however, laying insidious claim to a rival way of knowing subsumes the medical other into the learned physician's discourse, thereby appropriating that to which his rivals can no longer lay exclusive claim. Hart's learned profession is, in other words, in large measure fashioned by the paradox of a logos as argumentatively open to the competition as it is stalwart in its refusal to acknowledge grounds for reconciliation with or rhetorical concession to the empirics he so clearly disdains.

Though his dual status might also count him as one "of this stamp" that Hart includes among the empirics, physician–surgeon Edward Edwards makes it equally clear that rapprochement is not his concern. From the beginning of his 1636 *The Analysis of Chyrurgery*, Edwards thwarts any expectations of conciliation as he points an accusing finger at the suspect practices that define a medical "iron" age full of "imps" and "wretches." Inscribing a rhetorical divide that may fall along lines different from Hart's but is no less divisive or insistent, Edwards responds to what Sherwood calls "the calumnies of these times" ("To the Worshipfull *Alexander Read*" n. pag.) as he rails against the "posturing" and "diabolicall devices" of empirical offenders patently guilty of "impudent boasting" as well as the "disdainfull mocking" of those who are clearly their intellectual superiors. The learned may be free to overreach with impunity, as Hart's hyperbolic rhetoric in itself suggests, but the healers Edwards complains about deploy a suspect rhetoric that proves them nothing but "complainers, false accusers," and "dissembling hypocrites" (*Analysis* Sig. B_r/1). Edwards thus deploys a logos relying not on the evidence of careful reasoning but on assertions of rhetorical abuse aiming not to correct but appeal to a like-minded and already persuaded audience.

Edwards proves more attentive to the persuasion of reason in his 1637 *The Cure of All Sorts of Fevers*, where his epistle "To the friendly Reader" proceeds from the proposition that the healing arts "farre exceed all other faculties" to conclude that the "Repayrers of our sick, sore, and decayed bodies" therefore require "one skillful in that Profession" (*Fevers* Sig. $A2_r$). Though here not indulging in some rhetorical abuses of his own, Edwards proves no more interested than Hart in acknowledging what his hybrid profession might share with others; rather, it is by the incompetence of alternative healers, he insists, that "the thrice worthy and needful faculties of Physick and Chirurgerie are abused" (*Fevers* Sig. A2$_r$). Uniting abstract knowledge with the hands-on practice targeted by numerous physicians, however, Edwards aims not to separate "Physick and Chirurgerie," as Hart would have it, but to elevate the surgeon's qualifications to equal those of learned medicine. Much as Hart rhetorically appropriates and thus lays discursive claim to that of the empirical other, Edwards subsumes and therefore subordinates the surgeon's practice into the higher calling of learned medicine. It is "neither fit nor lawfull for every ignorant person that practiseth Chirurgery," he insists, without also commanding "that deep thrise worthy learned faculty of Physicke" (*Analysis* Sig. B2$_r$/3). Edwards's logos nevertheless relies on asserting the distinctiveness essential to defining any profession, a position he elsewhere makes clear in his insistence that a builder exceeds the capacity of a tailor or weaver to construct a house (*Fevers* Sig. A2$_r$). Edwards, in other words, is no less intent than Hart on fashioning a professional who may incorporate one calling into another but remains distinctly apart from all those medical others who prove useful only in defining by contrast the true professional he represents. Whether as loosely identified as Edwards's encompassing inclusion of all those who "boldly adventure on all the parts of physicke" without the physicians' learning (*Analysis* Sig. B2$_r$/3) or as specifically as they are in Hart's list, their unlearned rivals serve persuasive purpose as a largely undifferentiated mass of collective offence.[8]

The age-defining impishness Edwards laments becomes even more encompassing in Sir Thomas Browne's attack on "Saltimbancoes, Quacksalvers, and Charlatans." A work that professes by reason to challenge many "commonly presumed TRUTHS" attributed to science, natural philosophy, history, scripture, and medicine, *Pseudodoxia Epidemica* nevertheless indulges a heated ad hominem assault on those who mislead their subjects "not onely unto pecuniary defraudations, but the irreparable deceit of death." Such fraudulent practitioners are, Browne complains, akin to "Fortune tellers, Juglers, Geomancers, and the like incantatory impostors"

[8] Alison Klairmont Lingo ascribes similar rhetorical strategies to the two French physicians who wrote and published objections to alternative practitioners. Examining "how university-trained physicians presented their competitors as a medical 'other'" both "morally and professionally unfit to practice medicine" (583), Lingo underscores the French physicians' like "desire to eliminate economic competition" and points to their shared "anxieties about class, sexual, religious, and professional boundaries" (584). Like their English counterparts, the French physicians "enlisted their own religious beliefs, superstitions, and male support to convince their readers not to seek medical help from such dangerous characters" (584), finding a means to "achieve their goals" in the Reformation's "rhetoric of 'order'" (583).

who "betray the cause of truth" and "incensibly make up" a misleading and "legionrie body of errour" whose finer distinctions collapse into a single, opposing other (*Pseudodoxia* Sig. $B2_r$–$B2_v$/11–12; book 1, ch. 3). Appearing also in the *Religio Medici*'s description of "a traditional magick, not learned immediately from the devil, but at second hand from his scholars," the collective necromantic "body of errour" is thus "able and do empirically practise without his advice" (*Religio* 22; part 1, sec. 31). Browne's reference to those who "empirically practice" at least alludes to the unlearned medical practitioners he takes to task in *Pseudodoxia*, and his complaint that the devil's disciples cloak their knowledge of "the secret betrayed" under the guise of "traditional magick" more than suggests that empirical practitioners are no different from the equally conflated "incantatory imposters," for "both proceeding upon the principles of nature," Browne confirms, will "under any master, produce their effects" (*Religio* 22; part 1, sec. 31). Like Edwards and Hart, Browne claims for his profession a distinctiveness diametrically opposed to a conflation of medical rivals whose shared, erroneous ways of knowing are confirmed by the availability of effects open to "any master" among them.

The empiric thus serves as a broad catch-all category that may lack consistent definition but is of categorical usefulness to the logos of the physicians' arguments. Regardless of the combinations and kinds of differences physicians and writers as varied as Hart, Edwards, and Browne do (or do not) emphasize in defining themselves over against the empirical other, however, their self-fashioning rhetoric is nevertheless consistent in deploying a logos that insistently upholds the overriding, primary distinction of learned and lay. Their unlearned rivals, who are "altogether strangers to good education in the liberall Arts & Sciences" (2), as Hart puts it, lack the physician's learning, a necessity Andrew Boorde long before made clear in *The Breviarie of Health,* first published in 1547.[9] In addition to the trivium, Boorde asserts, the ideal physician needs not only natural philosophy, but also geometry, arithmetic, and astronomy, the latter "to know, how, when, and at what time everye medicine ought to bee ministred." Once these are mastered, he says, the student is "apt to studie phisick by speculation" and,

[9] Medicine's distaste for empirics, Stephen Pender explains, was first expressed in Plato's *Phaedrus*, where "Socrates insists that a rhetor must shun mere 'empirical routine' and, like a physician, cultivate natural talent (physis), knowledge (epistēmē), and practice (meletē)" ("Medicine and Rhetoric" 45). From the sixteenth-century adoption of Thomas Linacre by the College of Physicians, however, the medical curriculum had largely shunned the latter; as Reginald Magee points out, the first step in obtaining a medical degree was the trivium-oriented Bachelor of Arts, which required candidates to defend in Latin their knowledge of grammar, logic, and rhetoric (272).

on the basis of learning both intently bookish and theoretical, only then "boldlie a man may practice" (n. pag.). Given their lack of such "good education" (Hart, *Diet* 2), the unlearned are ill equipped to engage in the higher-order reasoning claimed by learned medicine's speculative epistemology and, though many physicians follow Galen in at least acknowledging some value in experience, it is useful only in conjunction with and is always subordinate to the learning acquired apart from and in preparation for practice.[10]

Accordingly, English's translation of *Galen's Method* resists the popularizing movement the vernacular purports to address and the practical turn the title page proclaims. Upholding the value of reason over observation, the Second Book of the work proper concludes that "all Method of Physick goes on as being separated from experience" and warns "those who study experience" therefore not to "undertake things above their reach." Avoiding such "great hazard," Galen's proffered theory ensures that otherwise experientially trained healers "would not omit and passe by those things which otherwayes they might understand." The knowledge "acquired by experience" and "such things as be only found out by reason" are different in both degree and kind, and it thus follows that "it is not to be admitted that those things should be mixed together." Observation may have its place, *Galen's Method* argues, "But seeing both of them are to be handled severally," experience and knowledge must only "be joined one after another." Upholding the humanist faith in reason over sense, the translation soon invokes Plato's insistence on the folly of inferring from

[10] Axtell explains that "throughout most of the seventeenth century the medical curriculum of Oxford and Cambridge was one of the most conservative in Europe because it remained, in the face of the clinical advances of Sydenham, the physiological breakthrough of Harvey, and the solid achievements of Lower, Willis, and the iatrochemical physicians, primarily a literary study of medicine" in which "Galen and Hippocrates continued to serve as "the main fare of the curriculum" (146). Sydenham, notes Cook, accrued "a reputation as the true English Hippocrates" and, though licensed by the London College of Physicians, "had strong antiacademic sentiments, believing that medicine ought to be taught by apprenticeship, not by books" (*Medical Regime* 185). Yet the physicians' modicum of non-textual training, which included witnessing an autopsy or two over the course of a medical degree, can also be read textually. As Stephen Pender concludes in response to Jonathan Sawday's study of dissection and anatomy, "one might claim that anatomical dissection itself is merely the visual culmination of discursive and recursive, 'thick' and rhetorical descriptions of embodiment" ("Interiority" 237), thus serving more to reinforce than complement their persistently bookish epistemology. Quoting Paul Feyerabend's remark that "different 'forms of life' have a different fate when put in the same surroundings, and some of them fare badly in the eyes of their own practitioners," Harley instead argues that "there is therefore no need to separate the construction of medical practice from that of theory. Medical knowledge is not merely representational; it is always praxis" ("Social Construction" 414). Harley may very well be right, but there is little question the learned physicians articulated a discursive view of medical practice that consistently privileged theory over practice.

worldly evidence ever variant and mutable. Presenting only a cheap, shadowy, or even patently false imitation of truth and not the higher abstracted knowledge of the learned physician, the evidence of experience must be kept vigilantly distinct lest it supersede or replace reason, for "invention is the knowledge of the disease itself" (*Galen's Method* 29), not what might be misguidedly or falsely inferred from its many manifestations. In dual and conflicting impulses that, on the one hand, aim to enable the practical efforts of "any judicious man" in expressed intent and, on the other, strive in the translation proper to privilege the learned physician's persistently theoretical orientation, the difference that lies between text and translator renders the whole of English's *Galen's Method* as open and distinctive as the rhetoric that defined early modern medicine.

The physicians thus acknowledge the value of greater experience when it suits their rhetorical purposes, as in Sherwood's contrasting of College members with the "small experience" of those "new beginners in the practice of Physick," but warn against its practical acquisition and application. Ironically, the harm done by the unlearned practitioner's experiential reliance cannot be redressed even by books themselves. Cotta, for instance, may acknowledge that books can be "paper-Apothecary-shoppes of secrets and medicines" (a statement in itself difficult to read positively, given his loathing of all things empirical), but insists they are at best useless and harmful without the physician's reason and wisdom. Such books therefore need be kept under wraps, "lest in ignorant handling and unwotting abuse their faire promising seemings prove gilded poysons" (Sig. D4_r–D4_v/ 23–24). Cotta's dual critique is both discursively and practically aimed, taking on both the "paper-Apothecary-shoppes" of medical information that might be useful in learned hands and the "gilded poysons" to which the medical other will surely transmute them. Without the learned physician's capacity for higher-order reasoning, Cotta argues, what might be good and useful becomes mere dross disguised under gold's thin veneer. Defining the physician's learning in contrast with the poisonous ignorance of unlearned rivals, Cotta's metaphor makes a very sharp distinction between his epistemology and theirs.

Not all are so vividly *enargeiac* in voicing their objections. Hart marks the divide in less inflammatory and more literal terms, defining the empiric as "especially unfurnished of that skil and sufficiency required in the practice of this so sacred and sublime profession of Physicke" (2). Given that the "sacred and sublime" true practice of physic transcends the quotidian, the earthly, and the concrete of a practical medicine assumed to stand in contrast, however, the rhetoric of Hart's professional self-fashioning is no less divisive if less divisively expressed. Browne also relies on a more tempered and less self-aggrandizing logos in defining his professional self by what it is not: "I am not of Paracelsus's mind," he writes in *Religio Medici*, "that boldly delivers a receipt to make a man without conjunction." In a work shaped by uncertainty, Browne is far less adamant than the vehement Cotta or the proselytizing Hart. Willing to question the grounds of the physician's way of knowing, Browne "yet cannot but wonder at the multitude of heads that do deny traduction, having no other arguments to confirm their belief than that rhetorical sentence and antimetathesis of Augustine, '*creando infunditur, infundendo creatur.*'" Such unquestioning subscription to "rhetorical sentence" leaves his *religio* untroubled, for "Either opinion," he reasons, "will consist well enough with religion," yet his *medici* need interrogate Augustine's superficially clever, chicken-and-egg tautology of "infused in creating, and created in infusing" offered in inherently circular antimetabolic form.[11] Browne may expressly reject the Paracelsian, but this does not make him a disciplinary hardliner; on the contrary, "I should rather incline," he writes, to that which is "not wrung from speculations and subtleties" of the kind that are presumably Galenic. Acknowledging the value of one's own experience, he would prefer instead to infer "from common sense and observation" and therefore rely on that "not pick'd from the leaves of any author, but bred amongst the weeds and tares of my own brain" (*Religio* 26; part 1, sec. 36). Inclining toward an epistemology we now understand as scientific empiricism but unable wholly to embrace it, the persistent ambivalence of Browne's tentatively wrought logos attests to the extent to which learned medicine's theory-privileging habits of thought were entrenched in early modern medical thinking.

Upholding the knowledge of abstracted understanding over that gleaned from experience or "the weeds and tares" of one's own brain, the physicians' arguments also reflect the longstanding debate between philosophy and rhetoric. In an intellectual context whose foundations had long rested on the trivium, what is theoretical aligns with the higher-order reasoning claimed by philosophy, whose part the humanist physicians take also by distancing themselves from a pragmatic approach more readily aligned with rhetoric. Privileging philosophy even as they rely on rhetoric, the

[11] The figure, which sees words or their variant forms repeated in reverse order, is sometimes mistaken for chiasmus. Both involve repetition in reverse order, but chiasmus, Richard Lanham explains, implies "a more precise balance and reversal" and "antimetabole a looser" that does not require repetition of words in the same form (14).

physicians aim to align their professional sympathy with the former. As the physicians inscribe nebulous distinctions originally propounded by philosophers and rhetoricians who, like the physicians and their unlearned rivals, had always been in competition both epistemologically and practically, they highlight differences upheld more readily in theory than practice.[12] Just as Peter Mack's philosopher styled himself above the rival orator who is shown to have "no interest in the truth or in goodness but is cynically devoted only to victory" (2), the learned physician claims a capacity for higher-order reasoning upheld in marked contrast with the specious thinking of medical rivals.[13] Hart, for instance, disdains those empirical practitioners whose collective tendency to "abuse right reason" (*Diet* 2) opposes the right reasoning of the theory-privileging physicians, while Cotta insists that all medical "others," the "travellers" in particular, are rhetorical abusers to the extent that they persuade "credulous men, for their owne gaine, into their owne hands" (114). Primrose more explicitly takes philosophy's part, however, as he claims that the errors of the people "disturbe the right reason of curing" (Sig. $B3_r$) and rejects rhetoric with the insistence that "diseases are not cured with Eloquence" (3). All three, of course, make such claims while indulging in some eloquent manipulations of their own. The result is that the distinction between the theoretical, and hence more philosophical, epistemology of learned medicine and that of the experientially oriented, hands-on practitioner so often accused of rhetorical abuse belies the learned physician's own willingness to deploy whatever means of persuasion suits his professionalizing agenda.

The learned physician, Primrose writes, is not one "that knowes a little Greeke and Latine, or some other Science besides Physick." Instead, he needs to be "well instructed in the Rules of Physick, and well read in Galen

[12] The distinctions between logic and rhetoric were always slippery, and sometimes valorizing one demanded a potentially self-subverting defence of the other. This may have been especially true for invention: "It was not uncommon," Joan Gibson notes, "even for those most keenly aware of the differences between logic and rhetoric, to render logical invention a species of rhetorical invention, and to distinguish them chiefly on the grounds of the greater plainness and brevity of logical invention." Logic and rhetoric were, in other words, inescapably intertwined as theory and practice and as conjoined aspects of the humanist trivium. "Renaissance theory," Gibson goes on to observe, thus "never really divorced rational speech and logic itself from practical considerations of politics and the professions" (17). Other discussions of physicians' self-presentation imply such a connection. "In the 'antiquack' literature of the period," Cook notes, "it is not as much the treatments they used but their inner character and outward behavior that separated the physicians form the rest" ("Good Advice" 19). Thus the physicians styled themselves as wise counsellors akin to philosophers rather than sources of the practical knowledge associated with rhetoricians.

[13] Vying for customers in the academic marketplace of ancient Greece, "the philosopher," Mack explains, likewise "found it necessary to expose the inadequacy of the rhetorician's view of the world," and did so "to win pupils for his more esoteric and apparently less useful training" (2).

and Hippocrates" and therefore "understands thoroughly the Diagnostick, Prognostick, and Therapeutick parts" (3).[14] The ancient physicians retain their authority, but their learned successors are in Primrose's formulation held to stand with and not apart from the practices of diagnosis, prognosis, and treatment.[15] As much as the physicians acknowledged the importance of *praxis* while insisting on privileging the theory to which they laid sole and singular claim, their professional claim staking was also served by their command of the "little Greeke and Latine" Primrose dismisses. The physicians' self-fashioning, in other words, was enabled by their knowledge of languages vernacular and ancient and, especially, by the rhetorical expertise that came with it. In his 1651 paratextual tribute to Primrose's newly translated treatise, Richard Roper points to the significant advantages granted by intensive study "in the liberall Arts & Sciences" made clear in expressed gratitude to the author who originally "spake to the *Learned*, not to *Vulgar* men" (n. pag. lines 1–2). Roper holds high hopes for those who

> Now in their proper Idiome they may see
> The Pop'lar Errours which in Physick be
> So Thou'rt the peoples guide, and foe to all
> Who do seduce by th'Art Empyricall:
> For now the strange delusions of that sect
> In English to all eyes thou do'st detect.
> (n. pag. lines 3–8)[16]

According to Roper, an ignorant public needs to be educated against empirical seduction, and the university-educated physicians are uniquely qualified for the job.

At the same time, the physicians' competence in Latin and ancient Greek that granted them control over learned medicine's most canonical

[14] Ian Maclean points out that Galen regarded "medical education" as "a craft apprenticeship" with "both a theoretical and a practical dimension," and that he valued the senses "to claim that there is a distinction between true and false which is necessary to any knowledge; and there are things evident to the senses and intellect" discernible through sight (255). Though undoubtedly aware of the position Maclean articulates, there seems little question that the physicians privileged the theoretical over the practical, the intellect over the senses.

[15] Proposing that physicians forgo the ancients by ignoring their practice and harkening only to their words, Richard Bunworth's *The Doctresse: A Plaine and Easie Method, of Curing Those Disease Which Are Peculiar to Women* (1656) offers a more extensive account of a professional ideal that acknowledges the importance of one's present senses in discovering knowledge (78–81). Physician–surgeon Edwards shares Bunworth's view but is more explicit with a subtitular *Theorique and Practique part thereof* uniting the Galenic and practical explicitly, philosophy and rhetoric implicitly. Edwards's practical interests are further confirmed by the numerous treatments and remedies offered in *The Cure of All Sorts of Fevers* (1637).

[16] The poem, "To his kind friend Dr. Wittie, upon his Translation of the Popular Errours," appears among a number of prefatory tributes.

texts allowed them to produce some equally inaccessible works of their own. In penning an argument intended not "to treate of the controversies of Physicians," Primrose suggests that he aims not to take up the physicians' internal debates. On the contrary, he intends "but onely to shew forth certain *Errours* of the people" (B3). Claiming not a specialist but popular topic, the book was nevertheless penned in a language inaccessible to the very offenders it aimed to correct. Hence the work itself is to some extent an overly laboured inside joke, a self-validating manifesto useful only to the colleagues its learned language included. Predicated in large measure on linguistic knowledge commanded by the educated professional he represents, Primrose's insistently exclusionary logos served merely to confirm what his like-minded colleagues already knew; hence the *Popular Errors* becomes a self-consuming artifact significant in its resolute failure to do what it proposes.[17] In rendering the original Latin of the *Popular Errors* into English, then, physician–translator Witty compromised the very distinctiveness both the original author and his translation aimed to uphold.

In his 1612 *A Short Discoverie*, Cotta instead professes to write "for the meanest readers sake," and has therefore "suited the plainnes and simplicitie of a familiar style" to the capacity of his intended audience. For those not conversant in the classical languages and "for facilitie of common reading," he has in the interests of his audience "smoothed and cleared the streame and current of this little volume" so as not to subject the reader unschooled in Latin or Greek to "the flops and interruptions of unusuall sounds and language" ("To the Reader" Sig. $A3_v$). A vernacular translation in Primrose's case and a plain English text in Cotta's are rhetorical necessities, an *exigence* demanding that the physicians' discourse be rendered accessible to the popular and rival audiences they meant also to exclude. Yet, as with English's translation of Galen, accommodation required that the physicians also subvert the linguistic mystique crucial to a profession whose logos depended on illustrating as well as upholding the differences between physicians and other kinds of medical practitioners as well as those duped by the common error.

[17] I borrow here, of course, from Stanley Fish's study of that title. I would argue that Primrose's treatise constitutes what Fish defines as "a rhetorical experience" to the extent that it too "can be placed and contained within the categories and assumptions of received systems of knowledge" (1). The received knowledge Primrose validates in an original accessible only to those who shared its assumptions, thus rendering the experience of reading as "flattering" as any "rhetorical form" (2) Fish identifies. In translation, Primrose's treatise offers the lay reader the "humiliating" experience of "dialectical form," succeeding for the learned physician as what Fish describes as "the vehicle" that persuades "at its own expense" (3).

Bound therefore to compromise their own arguments, the rhetorically savvy physicians are well aware of the problem, and are not averse to complaining about it. Hart, for one, opens his treatise with a disclaimer, making clear that he is compelled by duty and not desire metaphorically to take up the lesser occupation of the stage and speak openly of the physicians' exclusive right to the profession of medicine (*Diet* 1).[18] The physicians understand what rhetors and rhetoricians also know, that specialized discourse plays a crucial role in delineating and maintaining the bounds of any profession, and to speak outside those bounds is also to compromise them. Cotta's assertions of professional distinctiveness thus depend also on establishing the social, cultural, and intellectual advantages of a university education that, in both its distinctiveness and the rhetorical understanding it bestowed, went a long way in asserting as well as fashioning the physicians' authority. Even the licensed but experientially trained "Surgeons," reasons Cotta, have "neither letters nor humanity" and are not "acquainted with the dialect and language of the learned" (36) that facilitated the physicians' protectionist enterprise.

Emphasizing the surgeons' linguistic shortcomings in his sixteenth-century translation of Galen, Thomas Gale argued instead for advantages that would accrue "if the professors of Chirurgerie were learned in these tongues." One of only a few sixteenth-century surgeons "praised for their contributions to medical learning" (Cook, *Medical Regime* 46), Gale emphasizes what the surgeons ought to do rather than what they have neglected. An understanding of classical languages might, he argues, lead those lesser practitioners to "more easely understand the principles of their Arte, with their true divisions, and definitions" necessary to "readier instruct them to follow a true methode." In concert with his aim to improve the practice, Gale claims finding a "true method" in surgery as the "one cause which hath moved me to take this matter in hande" ("The Epistle Dedicatory" Sig. Aiv$_r$). Linguistic ignorance prevents the surgeons from attaining the standards of "true method," and Gale proposes a corrective that would see the surgeons rise to rather than be excluded from what he yet upholds as the physicians' higher-order professionalism. Whether advocating that others learn "these tongues," writing in a combination of Latin and English, or refusing to stoop to the vernacular, Gale, Hart, Cotta, and Primrose give voice to a contradiction that accommodates the physicians' reforming aims and their self-fashioning desires.

[18] Ironically, theatre also serves metaphorically for Primrose's bogus practitioners, the "Stage-Players" who are physicians in name but not performance (3).

The paradox that marks the rhetoric of learned medicine is thus very much the product of an *exigence* demanding arguments of distinctiveness that are undercut by the necessity of a plain vernacular yet fortified by the implication that the medical other need also rise to the physicians' level of learning. Though their professionalizing enterprise sometimes required the physicians to speak a discourse unsuited to their elite, learned status, the physicians also upheld their learned distinction in the manner of a delivery that, like Primrose's Latin, may have served a purpose less inclusive than their linguistic choices imply. Seeming also to address an audience already persuaded by his argument, Cotta advocates an appropriate correspondence of vernacular form and learned content in a "style," he notes in his dedication, that cannot be "so farre in love with it selfe as to forget the matter." It is crucial that the physicians' *elocutio* not be so lofty to compromise the exigence to which the logos of their arguments responds, and it is equally important that "brevity doth not suffer the reading" (Sig. $A2_v$) of a text whose form must also suit the gravitas of the problem it means to redress. Advocating a mean somewhere between the grandest and plainest, Cotta implies an elocutio inclined toward the expectations of the learned and therefore less open to the lay than the vernacular alone may suggest.

In a work accompanied by notes offered exclusively in Latin expressly intended for "refreshing onely the learned in the margine" ("To the Reader" Sig. $A3_v$), Cotta also renders the substance of his work even more fully accessible to those already the most capable of grasping it. Though professing an accommodating style in claiming to write in a broadly appealing way to a popular audience, to refresh only the learned in a paratextual language known to all physicians but not to all readers is to make visible at a mere glance the contradictory openness and distinctiveness evident throughout Cotta's treatise as a whole. Upholding the professional divide visually as well as verbally, the simultaneously inclusive and exclusive *dispositio* seen in the arrangement of a pointedly bifurcated page achieves a visible correspondence of form and content that mimicks in its ordering the larger distinction his argument upholds.[19] Though Hart's marginal

[19] Publishing medical works in English, Ted Brown notes, was spurred by an increasing esteem for the language, the vernacular shift protestantism entailed, and the desire of learned medicine to heighten its authority, making it more apparent and broadly recognized through greater accessibility. Hence "vernacular medical publication," Brown observes, functioned as a kind of "two-edged sword" in that "it provided a means for those on the lower levels of the medical scale to advance themselves at the expense of physicians" while "it also provided a means for those at the top to exert greater power over those below them" (106). Yet Cotta's concession to English in his text proper combined with the adherence to Latin in the marginal notes allows him to fashion his authority by drawing simultaneously on both the familiar and esoteric. Though not uncommon, the strategy allows an

gatekeeping differs from Cotta's in that he also offers occasional notes in English to accommodate the less-educated reader, he is not untroubled by the expressive limitations of argumentive *exigence*. In a later chapter on grief and sadness, for instance, Hart complains that those emotions have "diverse names in the ancient languages" but "by reason of the penury of our vulgar tongue," they "cannot all be Englished by severall termes" (*Diet* 393).[20] The limitations of a vernacular unable to express abstractions with precision, "the penury of our vulgar tongue," is at one with the intellectual limitations of a popular audience that cannot hope to achieve the physicians' capacity for higher-order reasoning.

Expressing disdain that has as much to do with class as education, Browne in his *Pseudodoxia Epidemica* complains of medical competition consisting of "men of inferiour ranke" (12; book 1, ch. 3) who lack formal education and whose undiscerning dupes are also of "lowe degrees" (11; book 1, ch. 3). Taking aim at the most scurrilous of his medical rivals, Browne insists on their incompetence in a response heated enough to confirm the very real threat of those lesser practitioners to the physician's hegemonic enterprise. In the preface of a document whose urgency of exigence is everywhere implied by an admittedly hurried tone, Browne states as much in apologizing for the less-than-ideal package in which his argument appears as he blames the distraction and demands of the profession he aims to defend,

> which though it leadeth us into many truths that passe undiscerned by others, yet doth it disturbe their communications, and much interrupteth the office of our pens in their well intended transmissions: and therefore surely in this wo[r]ke attempts will exceed performances: it being composed by snatches of time, as medi[c]all vacations, and the fruitless importunity of Vroscopy would permit us. ("To the Reader," *Pseudodoxia* n. pag.)

Browne's *apologia* is a telling one. Even though he wishes, like Primrose, to disabuse those who commit the common errors he identifies, his desire to communicate such offences is thwarted by the demands of a profession offering only "snatches of time" amidst "fruitless importunity." Browne was evidently too busy treating the stone that ran rife in his jurisdiction to devote proper attention to the argument he makes. His apology may

author both to "exert greater power" with the persuasive force of the vernacular and to preserve the mystique of the ancient.

[20] Writers from Thomas More onward sometimes championed English for reasons beyond accessibility. For a recent and thorough survey of the importance of "native eloquence" to a national identity defined by a uniquely English style and of the vernacular in rhetorical training and published handbooks, see Jenny C. Mann's *Outlaw Rhetoric* (Cornell University Press, 2012).

defend a profession disruptive of "well intended transmissions," but it is one that also leads to "many truths that passe undiscerned by others."

For Browne, the "many truths" uniquely accessible to the physician include his keener awareness, even when pressed, of rhetoric's uses and abuses. Yet those foolish enough to seek the help of medical interlopers are, he explains in *Pseudodoxia Epidemica*, universally deceived by their inability to discern mere persuasion from the logos of careful reasoning. "Thus unto them," he writes, "a piece of Rhetorick is a sufficient argument of Logick, an Apologue of A sope, beyond a Syllogisme in Barbara, parables then [sic] propositions, and proverbs more powerfull, then demonstrations" (*Pseudoxica* 8–9; book 1, ch. 3). The rhetorical problem Browne addresses points also to some pressing questions at the heart of the medical-epistemological debate, which had long asked how particular example and individual experience could help practitioners effectively negotiate what Stephen Pender describes as "the infinite diversity of human experience" ("Uncertainty" 15) medicine aims to address. An advocate of the newly inductive reasoning of science, Browne nevertheless recognizes the problems inherent in inferring universal rule from particular example, going on to note how the gullible are persuaded not by reason but "led rather by example, then precept, receiving perswasions from visible inducements, before intellectual instructions; and therefore also do they judge of humane actions by the event; for being uncapable of operable circumstances, or rightly to judge the prudenciality of affairs, they onely gaze upon the visible successe, and thereafter condemn or cry up the whole progression" (*Pseudodoxia* 9; book 1, ch. 3).

Browne thus remains dissatisfied in expressing the truths he aims to impart and laments his work's lack of rhetorical finesse. "And therefore also," he preemptively admits with a qualifying "perhaps," his treatise "hath not found that regular and constant stile, those infallible experiments, and those assured determinations, which the subject sometime requireth." Tellingly, though, it is precisely his profession that prohibits, and a more eloquent work "might be expected from others" who are not so busy seeking out the physician's "many truths," but "whose quiet doors and unmolested hours afford no such distractions" (*Pseudodoxia*, "To the Reader" n. pag.). Browne expresses here an interest more focused than most physicians on the importance of well-wrought language, a rhetorical sensibility evident also in the works that would bring about his literary renown. At the same time, he offers and accepts his rhetorical shortcomings as the inevitable by-product of a higher calling, making clear that "assured determinations" and "infallible experiments" in language cannot be expected from one who cannot separate his compulsion to write from his work as a healer and still fulfill his professional duties. Yet his proffered *litotes*, the figure of understatement that may aim more to bolster his profession than apologize for what his treatise lacks, suggests that his proclaimed rhetorical shortcomings are not exactly that. Considering that Browne is an especially admired prose stylist, such a supposition is at least in part verified by a disclaimer ingenuous in telling something quite different from what he elsewhere famously shows. Regardless of sincerity or intent, however, the hierarchy of value implied by Browne's elevating the duty of the physician over the compulsions of the rhetor suggests mixed feelings about the very tool that gives voice to his arguments, thus articulating the ambivalence that shapes the open yet distinctive rhetoric of early modern medicine more generally.

Though sometimes evident in their lamenting the rhetorical abuses of others while indulging in an abusive rhetoric of their own, the physicians' willingness to exploit while rejecting or devaluing the art of linguistic persuasion may be most insidious in an equally shared tendency to embrace rhetoric's advantages one moment and lament its shortcomings the next. Alluding to rhetorical usefulness in his discussion "Of the Empiricke," Cotta defends the physicians' book learning, maintaining that "there must needs be in all actions want of much more necessary knowledge then sense and experience canne advance unto." In doing so, he privileges the knowledge of a tradition that has always been intensely rhetorical. Even the "longest age," he goes on, cannot "so fully furnish and instruct in many things, as much more speedily doth prudent invention." The first of rhetoric's five canons Aristotle defines as finding the available means of persuasion, *inventio* also furnishes the self-persuasion that goes hand in hand with instructive possibility. As every early modern student's commonplace book can attest, the invention that facilitates understanding for both rhetor and auditor is most readily available from extant sources; as Cotta explains, it is "occasioned and helped by bookes and reading, which are both keyes unto all knowledge" (Sig. $C2_r$/11). In Aristotelian terms, such evidence falls under the rubric of invention's "nonartistic" or *atechnic* proofs. Sometimes known as "inartificial," it is the kind of evidence, often literary, that comes with a built-in argument. Typically for the Renaissance humanist, Cotta insists that genuine knowledge results not from experience but the written word that passeth worldly understanding.

Yet Cotta goes on to reason that books might also serve as a source of empirical knowledge. Professing that they are "rich storehouses of experiences, not onely of an age and countrie, but of all times & nations," Cotta champions reading over doing; simultaneously praising books as depositories of experience, however, he also undercuts the physicians' anti-empiric, anti-experiential arguments. If it arrives second-hand and serves the physicians' bookish orientation, though, what would otherwise be styled empirical is embraced as a desirable aspect of rhetorical practice: "Neither have I esteemed it any indecorum for the meanest understanding sake," Cotta writes in his address to the reader, "to insert particular cases and reports," *exempla* that are "neither least pleasing nor least profitable unto the vulgar."[21] But it turns out that Cotta invokes the *atechnic* primarily as "an inducement to reade, and an enticement to continue" (Sig. $A3_v$); in Cotta's hands, what is empiric serves the aims of verbal seduction rather than any demand for scientific proof. Rhetoric thus becomes not only the means by which the physicians pit themselves against the empirics, but also that by which the empirical is rehabilitated to fit the deeply textual epistemology of the university-trained physicians.

Evincing the humanist's awareness of Greene's two-faced coin, physicians also voice a mistrust of rhetoric that may equal their distaste for all things empiric. Such a paradoxical view Cotta conveys primarily through his critique of the kind of evidence on which the proof of logos may be based. Because they "glut the sense with stories of experiences past," he also says, books can also inhibit knowledge; hence neither one's own experience nor the recorded accounts of others have true epistemic value. Rather, Cotta insists that only "reason and judgement" can "truly enrich the mind, and give daily new increase and light in before untried & unexperienced truth" (Sig. $C2_r$/11). The ambivalence of self-contradiction soon becomes outright hostility when, despite his earlier heaping up of *exempla* for his readers' benefit, Cotta professes the inadequacy of such evidence in the hands of the rival empiric: "Example and imitation (which are the rules of an Apothecaries practice)," he insists, "are but patterns of anothers sufficiencie" (47). Later, Cotta again indicts rhetorical practice in exposing the "falsehood and lying imitation" (111) of travelling healers. Far from achieving the rhetorical virtue of *mimesis*, imitation in misguided hands becomes the enabler of charlatans. It is by deceptive mimicry, Cotta insists, that surgeons work "by lying promises, perswading many honest simple parents to commit their children" (36) to a bogus and inferior education. Surgical apprentices are thus sacrificed by parents

[21] As Stephen Pender notes, "medical reasoning relies on signs and examples, both gleaned from experience and both the subject of rhetorical inquiry; like rhetoric, medicine reaches plausible conclusions from probable premises" ("Medicine and Rhetoric" 39).

who may be honest but are of as "lowe degrees" as Browne's lamented dupes (*Pseudodoxia* 11; book 1, ch. 3).

Even physician–surgeon Edwards takes the physicians' part as he attributes the country surgeon's failings to a lack of formal education also aligned with social class.[22] Bemoaning the many abuses of others in his dedicatory epistle to the physician Alexander Read and the Company of London Surgeons, Edwards laments those who commit medical homicide "chiefly in the Country" (*Analysis* Sig. $B2_r/3$). The problem is, he writes, that those country surgeons have "neither conscience, learning, art ... nor never had good Tutor to instruct them" (Sig. $A2_v$). Invoking an analogy akin to English's insistence that working without Galen's guidance renders any medical practice as futile as "a blind man throwing his staffe at a dog" (n. pag.), Edwards argues that practical training alone is insufficient: "he that worketh without the perfect rules of the theoricke parts of this Art," he writes, "doth worke but as a blindman that caryeth a Picture: cutting sometimes too much, sometimes too little, as well, where hee should not, as where hee should, and so marres all" (*Analysis* Sig. $A3_r$).[23] As medical orthodoxy would have it, Edwards privileges the

[22] "In provincial towns and villages," Pelling and Webster observe, "the majority of practitioners" were "formally apprenticed," "not educated at a university," and "associated with gilds" (233), while Freidson points out that the physicians' elitist enterprise saw many alternative healers "driven out of practice or driven underground into the urban slums, the country side, and the cultist drawing room" (47). Physician Stephen Bradwell more clearly aligns the lesser country practitioner with beliefs about class in his epistle "To All That Have Cause to Love London," where he addresses those who possess "faire Houses, rich Furniture, delicious Fare, and curious cloathing; yea your full content" and advises that in the midst of plague those "that are Rich" need stay "to helpe the Poore." Accordingly, those should also remain "that have tru skill in Physicke to helpe the sicke," while those who are "Mountebancks" ought instead "quack in the Country among the contemners of Learning" (*Physick for the Sicknesse* Sig. A3v). That the "physicians sought clients and patrons likely sympathetic to their views," as Harley notes, may imply that Bradwell's physician is encouraged to remain among the prosperous to facilitate the patronage that was, says Harley, "a crucial method of mitigating or circumventing market competition." If "successful cognitive styles in medicine were those suited to either patronage or the marketplace" ("Social Construction" 414), as Harley claims, then class also worked to shape the profession of the medical elite. That early modern medicine was in other ways political Elmer confirms in his discussion of medicine and politics, where he finds "further evidence for the growing politicisation of medicine and the medical profession during the course of the seventeenth century" that "can be found in the ever-growing numbers of medical men who were willing to stand for public office." Medicine's politicization was manifest at every level, beginning with the local, where "physicians, surgeons and apothecaries increasingly served as the mayors of corporations, while countless others stood as burgesses or aldermen," and others "performed valuable service as justices of the peace in their localities." Even "at national level," elite practitioners became increasingly involved as "a number of physicians were elected to Parliament" ("Politics of Healing" 234).

[23] Hence physician–surgeons like Lancelot Coelson argue "Art" will only be "weak without practice" (*The Poor-Mans Physician and Cyrurgion* [1656], "To the Reader" n. pag.). According to Bernard Capp's *DNB* entry, Coelson "provided sensible guidelines and details of 300 medical recipes," but

humanist training that was the cornerstone of every learned physician's education and could be claimed also by physician–surgeons like him; at the same time, however, he expresses an epistemological allegiance more closely allied with practical medicine as he exhorts his readers "with all diligence to search out the secrets of nature, and endeavour chiefly hereby to stir up Gods glory" (*Analysis* Sig. E_r/25).

Invoking rival and presumably irreconcilable epistemologies to prove a counter argument, the physicians' rhetoric proves as specious as those they claim to argue against. Yet the differences between the physician's theory and the surgeon's praxis were no doubt exacerbated by allegiances to long-standing habits of thought whose distinctions became exaggerated in the face of practical medicine's growing popularity. At the same time, James Bono explains, even the chemical practice of a physician like Paracelsus, who famously called for the end of "the Age of Bookish culture," could not utterly free itself from the Galenic physicians' influence any more than the physicians proved capable of denying his. Given that, as Bono puts it, Paracelsian medicine promoted the idea that "nature is itself a 'book,' every page of which bears the unmistakable imprint – 'signature' – of the divine," even the most empirically oriented of physicians depended on reading out of a text metaphorical and therefore ever subject to interpretation. In a context where medicine, religion, and rhetoric are always to some degree inseparable, the necessity of reading the signs of nature is inextricably connected with the work of the religious exegete, signifying as it does what Bono describes as "a profound engagement with the *verbum Dei* and with the problem of how humans may gain access to it" (129).[24] Hence reading out of texts natural and divine through worldly evidence is as crucial to the fashioning of Edwards's ideal professional as it is to Hart's overreaching physician, both uniquely equipped to search out nature's secrets along with those of the ancients on whom they equally predicated their medical authority. Only he who has mastered the "perfect rules of the theoricke parts of this Art," Edwards thus insists in his opening epistle to Alexander Read, can avoid "cutting sometimes too much, sometimes

his work was "based on traditional galenical principles." Perhaps predictably by the 1668 publication of his "alchemical work Philosophia maturata," however, Coelson had "come to adopt Paracelsian principles."

[24] Paracelsus's "Doctrine of Signatures," Katherine Knight explains, surmised that "God had mercifully ensured that something about the plant had an affinity with a particular disorder or organ." Hence "lungwort, with spotted leaves suggesting pulmonary disease, could be used to cure chest complaints" while "plants with yellow flowers, or yellow spices, might be good for jaundice" (240).

too little" in the way that only a true artist can produce a worthy painting (*Analysis* Sig. $A3_r$).[25]

Reminiscent of Philip Sidney's famous borrowing from Horace, that the "speaking Picture" can teach as well as delight and his parallel (and professionalizing) insistence that, as Sidney suggests, "the first and most noble sort" of poets "range onely reined with learned discretion" (*Defence* 15), Edwards's metaphor invites a connection made explicit in a treatise that actually mentions the revered poet–martyr who was also among the most accomplished of English rhetors and rhetoricians.[26] In the address "To the Reader" that follows, Edwards not only further implies a class-conscious view in his admiration for the aristocratic Sidney, but also invokes the poet's authority to complain of those who would choose distinctiveness over openness. Those who refuse to share their knowledge, Edwards insists, act in the interests of intellectual (and presumably economic) protectionism and therefore "lovingly linke in league with the devil." Interested only in that which feeds their "filthy fancies," those with such "obstinate wils" and "barren fruitlesse hearts" also "swell with intolerable pride and envy" and "participate not with that worthy renowned knight, Sir *Philip Sidney*, who said love them that doe some good, because there be many that doe none at all" (*Analysis* B_v–$B2_r$/2–3). Reminded by Sidney of the Christian duty exemplified in Matthew's parable (25.14–30), "let such take heed," Edwards goes on, "that they perish not with such as hide their talent." Professing instead to leave "some fruits of my labours to posterity," Edwards further reminds his reader that Hippocrates and Galen insisted that healing knowledge must be used and perhaps also shared (*Analysis* B_v–$B2_r$/2–3).[27] Akin to a preacher in a pulpit, Edwards invokes the logos

[25] Thomas Blount makes a similar claim in his 1654 *Academy of Eloquence*: "The conceits of the mind are pictures," he writes, "whose Interpreter is the tongue" (Sig. A2v), while Stephen Pender reminds us of the metaphor appearing also in Thomas Wilson's paraphrase of Quintilian " 'Rhetorique at large paints wel the cause' which logic speaks in 'but a worde' " ("Medicine and Rhetoric" 63).

[26] Sidney is credited with penning the first work of literary criticism in English and is also cited in early modern rhetorics, not only in the fifty-two references found throughout Abraham Fraunce's 1588 *Arcadian Rhetorick*, but also in Blount's handbook (1, 5, and 10) and John Smith's 1673 *The Mysterie of Rhetorick Unveil'd* (147).

[27] Hart alludes to the parable also in the introduction to his epistle "To the Right Honorable Edward Lord Montague," where he likens himself to Diogenes, who refused to retire to "rest and ease," but insisted on running his philosophical race even as "he drew to the end thereof." Hart has likewise "not hid my talent in a napkin" by "keeping within mine owne breast that knowledge I had both in the University, and by many yeeres experience acquired in the profession of Physicke." On the contrary, Hart claims to have "endevoured to bee profitable to this present age" as well as "to propagate some directions to posterity" (*Diet* n.p).

of religious belief to persuade an audience whose attentiveness to scripture might be matched by reverence for the inimitable yet aspirational Sidney.

As might be expected, the physicians' debate with the empirics depended less on religion than their arguments with the physician–clerics. Edwards is not, however, the only treatise writer to invoke scripture in dispute with other rivals. Browne, for instance, makes the connection between the Fall and the "popular errors" he identifies in as its first cause (*Pseudodoxia* Sig. b_r), while Cotta's complaint against the empirics sometimes draws on the logos of scripture to launch a diatribe against women. As early modern writers of all kinds are wont to do, Cotta invokes the Genesis story as he laments that "Old Eve will never be worne out of Adams children." Renaissance writers never tire of citing the first human story, and they do so most often with the aim of confirming woman's grievous faults and the dangers inherent in the language that persuaded Adam to transgress in the first place. Oddly, though, Cotta implies that he might use the biblical account to defend as he maintains that "an apple" can in effect "do no great hurt." In a surprisingly positive spin on Genesis 3, Cotta even begins to sound like one of Eve's champions (Aemilia Lanyer's "Eves Apologie" springs readily to mind),[28] as he goes on to reason that the fruit "is faire and beautifull unto the eye, pleasant to taste, and but a trifle, a small matter, a little quantity, and of excellent quality Adam must needs taste." In keeping with his larger topic, Cotta even introduces medicinal possibilities inferred from the fruit's sensible virtues. The apple, he writes, "is an excellent medicine to make him see," for it "is good for his eyes" and "will cleare his sight" (Sig. $E3_v$/30).

Cotta's musings end with a leading *erotema*. "What is more faire, more easie, more gentle, more harmelesse, more cordiall, more daintie then an apple?" he poses in a rhetorical question heaped also with a comparative *diacope* imbuing the repeated "more" with the force of insistent repetition.[29] Cotta, of course, goes on to answer his own question, surmising that "Eve in good will offered it, and so Adam tooke it" and "It make him also see" (Sig. $E3_v$/30). Promising it may seem that Eve acted in "good will," but that Cotta twice invokes Adam's new-found ability to "see" also anticipates the forthcoming confirmation that the senses

[28] Lanyer's 1611 *Salve Deus Rex Judaeorum*, a poetic retelling of Christ's passion, features the wife of Pontius Pilate voicing a defence of women predicated on Eve's good will in offering Adam the knowledge men have subsequently claimed. For an extensive rhetorical reading of the poem, see Bennett, *Women Writing of Divinest Things*.

[29] Burton categorizes diacope as a "Figure of Pathos" (*Silva Rhetoricæ*), and there is no denying the emotional appeal of the Fall to a Christian audience.

ultimately deceive and Eve's proffered apple is therefore much less than a good thing. Foreshadowed by a perhaps-sarcastic repetition, the *ironia* of rhetorical questions already undone by an understood, anti-empirical mistrust of the senses would not escape the discerning reader, who would likely also anticipate the forthcoming change of tune. Sounding more like an unqualified assertion than the seductive yet recognizably specious reasoning that precedes it, Cotta's argument closes by confirming that the sight Adam gains, as every seventeenth-century reader would know, comes at terrible cost: "but Adam," he laments, "had bene better still blind," for "a dangerous and incurable leprosie and infection thence seised upon him, which after none but the great Physition of heaven and earth could cure" (Sig. $E3_v$/30). The Fall may have offered access to otherwise-forbidden knowledge but also cut humanity irrevocably off from the most important of all, the knowledge of the divine that remains "ever secret" and "ever beyond itself" (Foucault, Intro.). Invoking the familiar logos of scriptural exegesis, Cotta replicates the seductive potential of both language and women, and preemptively clinches his conclusion that women are a species of anti-healer, unfit to practise healing and the harbingers of diseases that may be metaphorical but are beyond the capacity of any to relieve let alone cure.

Taken up in numerous medical treatises, the topic of women is especially prevalent in those that are, like Cotta's, preoccupied with issues of professionalism. In Cotta's formulation, the divine Word itself discredits the domestic healers who may not be the most obvious but were the most deeply entrenched of the physicians' many medical competitors.[30] Confirmed by the story so often invoked to prove woman's oft-iterated inferiority, her primal culpability also renders her among the most dangerous of medical interlopers. The damage they inflict may be the worst of all, and such "*Women Physicians*," as Hart sarcastically dubs them (*Diet* 2), also prove the worst of unqualified meddlers. Claiming hard evidence to prove women ill equipped for healing, Hart goes on to describe the ill-doings of a certain "Pettie-coat Physitian" whose many "blisterings" resulted in harms so numerous they are "too tedious" to recount and therefore not

[30] Cotta's discourse is, of course, hyperbolic. Many early modern women practised healing quite successfully and unchallenged while Cotta and other physicians fashioned a context in which they could assert their authority with indignation and vitriol. What recent scholarship has taught us, cautions Fissell, is "that the outrage expressed by physicians and surgeons about female healers must be understood as situational," a piece of the larger rhetorical agon I explore here and what she describes as "specific interventions in longer-term campaigns of self-fashioning and self-promotion" ("Introduction" 8).

even necessary to an argument that really needs no making.[31] Unlearned and thus unable "to dive into the depth of the true causes," writes Hart, the petticoat practitioner "must needs be ignorant of the true cure" that might even elude the genuine healer: "And this being a taske which often poseth the most skilfull Artist in his profession," Hart *erotemically* asks, "what then should we expect from such a she-Physitian?" (*Diet* 10).

Complaining of "petticoat *Physitians* and Chyrugians" as well as "those Male-kinde" he dubs "caterpillars," Edwards laments the dangers of their invasive and "huge swarme." Lacking any real knowledge or training, petticoat healers are mere "tatling gossips," though their homebound role means they are also "frequent among sicke folks." Hence "hearing the advice and counsell of the learned and expert Physitian," women are also privy to his "prescribing many fit things to his Patient." Typically seizing opportunity to grasp knowledge above their reach, such "audacious gossips" presume to "give syrups, senæ, Rubarb, Cassia, Manna, Aloes, &c. and not onely clysters, but also strong purges, and vomits" that, Edwards insists, prove "no more fit for the disease, but by chance." Practising by uninformed mimicry, women are in league with the worst of the empirics who, like the cobbler aiming "to make shoes fit for every mans foot upon one Last," are just as likely to miss the mark. Aspiring to meet what ignorance makes impossible to achieve, such "idle wretches" lack even the capacity to recognize how little they know. "If these learned faculties were so easily attained," Edwards insists, one might expect others also to recognize "that men would never bestow so long time and great charges in studie, and learning to attain the [physician's] deepe knowledge." Railing at the presumption of "this godless crue," Edwards champions the learned physican far above those who presume "to minister medicines from so slender a ground-worke" (*Analysis* Sig. $A3_r$).

As much as Cotta, Edwards, and Hart may berate the petticoat practitioner, Primrose does them one better in foregrounding, both visually and verbally, his assault on women healers. Leaving no doubt about the book's primary target, the frontispiece of the Witty translation depicts a sick man with a physician, an angel, and a woman at his bedside. Explicated in verse on the facing page, the illustration features a woman who "comes in *charitie* / To see the sicke and brings her *remedie*" (n. pag., lines 1–2), a "*pepper posset*" unavailable in any "'*Pothecaries* shoppe" yet claimed to cure "Fever, Strangury, and Stone" (lines 10–12). Though the woman believes her

[31] Edwards uses "Petticote Surgeons" (*Analysis* Sig. A2v) to describe the women practising medicine who were also derisively referred to as "petticoat doctors."

remedy to be "of more desert / Then all *Hippocrates*, or *Galens* Art" (line 18), the patient needs rescue from her unorthodox ministrations. Behind her is thus "an *Angell*" who "gently puts her backe," and "Lest such *erroneous* course the sicke doe wracke," instead "Leads the *Physitian*, and guides his hand" (lines 19–21). The angel "approves his *Art*, and what he doth must stand," for it is his "*Art* that God allowes," and the physician only "by him 'tis blest / To cure disease, leave then all the rest" (lines 22–24).

Primrose champions the divinely sanctioned "*Art*" of the poem's closing couplet and reiterates his critique throughout his treatise. Disputing the value of homemade possets and other traditional remedies in chapter after chapter, Primrose tackles the female sex especially in his fifth, "Of Women that meddle in Physick and Surgery," where he complains that "they usually take their remedies out of English books, or else make use of such as are communicated to them by others," describing in the process the written and oral transactions of a discourse community whose knowledge and methods – its defining logos, in other words – ran contrary in application as well as vernacular origin to those of the learned physician. Hence Primrose advises against strict adherence to the specifics of a given receipt the medical manuals propose. Insisting instead that responsible treatment is always context dependent, for "*Galen* in his bookes of *Method* teaches that remedies are to bee altered according to the person, place, part affected, and other circumstances" (20), he invokes ancient authority to prove his point. Like other physicians, Primrose advocates the application of right reason and the understanding of "true causes" to assess and address individual medical problems. Tellingly, the ability to adapt successfully and appropriately to a given situation is, of course, a skill necessary also to every capable rhetor.

In his tribute to the Witty translation, Andrew Marvell seems to imply that some women share that ability. In the poem's second stanza, Marvell commends one in particular:

> Celia whose English doth more richly flow
> Then Tagus, purer then dissolved snow,
> And sweet as are her lips that speake it, she
> Now learns the tongues of France and Italie;
> But she is Celia still: No other grace
> But her own smiles commend that lovely face;
> Her native beauty's not Italianated,
> Nor her chaste minde into the French translated:
> Her thoughts are English, though her sparkling wit
> With other language doth them fitly fit.
> Translatours learne of her.
>
> (n. pag. lines 17–27)

Commentators have noted that "Celia" may have been Marvell's tutee, Mary Fairfax, the Civil War general's daughter whose learning the poet elsewhere famously commends.[32] But the teacher–poet seems to have admired his subject also for her rhetorical skill, for she not only had mastered English, but also knew something of the art of using it well. Though Marvell's Celia has not learned Greek or Latin, the poet grants high praise in a work that is also one of few pieces of literary criticism we have from its author.

As much as he may profess to admire Celia, however, the poet seems interested in making visual as well as verbal distinctions between his facility with language and hers. Presented in bifurcated arrangement akin to Cotta's appending of Latin marginalia to vernacular text, the English version of Marvell's poem is preceded by a Latin counterpart that, in proving his ability to reason and write in the language of the ancients, also confirms the higher status he shares with the physicians. Celia's thinking, by contrast, is thoroughly and exclusively vernacular. Her skill with English may confirm her "native beauty" and "chaste minde," yet such praise seems rather backhanded if the classically trained poet really means to commend his subject's education, ability, and knowledge. Celia may possess a "sparkling wit" in her native tongue but, however effervescent that wit may be, she cannot move beyond the vulgar if she can neither speak nor reason in the ancient languages. Though the poet implies that she may have the potential to do so, for "*Translatours* learne of her," his assertion quickly becomes evidence of his own reason compromised. With a heavy midline caesura, the poet reclaims control to avoid sliding "Downe into *Errour* with the vulgar tide" (lines 27–28). The reality is that

> Women must not teach here: The *Doctor* doth
> Stint them to Cawdles, Almond milk, and broth.
> Now I reforme; and surely so will all
> Whose happy eyes on thy *Translation* fall.
> (lines 29–32)

Moving away from the topic of Celia, the poet enacts and avers what Primrose's book argues and Cotta's retelling of the Fall confirms, that the language of women must be resisted and, ultimately, governed by that of men – in this case, by the male physicians who are the only proper healers. Together with the "Now I reforme" insinuating that he may once have

[32] See "Upon Appleton House," lines 707–10.

thought differently about women's capacity to heal, the poet's praise and his competing impulses show how "the distinctions of knowledge" Wear claims "both exist and do not exist in English popularized medicine of this period" ("Popularization" 33) also parallel those that exist and do not exist between language and healing and between women and men.

Healers who wrote from beyond the pale were not, however, ambivalent in denying the distinctions of medical knowledge. The "A.M." of *A Rich Closet of Physical Secrets* (1652) lays claim to learned authority with substance drawn significantly from a "Phisitians Collections" and partly by the author "with his own hands from an antient Manuscript" ("To the Reader" Sig. $A2_r$). Shrewdly, A.M. both acknowledges the knowledge of the early modern physician and, by noting the "antient" status of the manuscript from which much of the book's content derives, recognizes the Galenic authority that had long distinguished learned medicine. But A.M., who may actually represent the "four severall Students in Physick" claiming authorship on the title page, in noting the manuscript "found in an Abby at their dissolution" also positions that knowledge in league with a tradition whose contemporary legitimacy came into being with the English Reformation. Allying the book with a protestant tradition more usually associated with Paracelsus and simultaneously claiming orthodox orientation, A.M.'s legitimizing claim may also imply a waning Galenic authority and a medical paradigm shift that was neither instantaneous nor complete. As much as other practitioners might acknowledge the authority of and even defer to the physicians' classical and textual epistemology, then, the medical elite remained on guard because, as A.M.'s cautious maneuvering suggests, no amount of deference could remove the threat of an ever-present other to their professional status.

That printed works on empirical and traditional medicine neither endorsed by the London College nor produced by its members were thriving by century's end may indicate that renegade and even irregular practitioners were indeed capable participants in the intensely rhetorical culture in which they lived and worked. Though most alternative practitioners lacked access to the level of education claimed by the physicians, the eventual success of alternative and once-unorthodox practices suggests that many of the physicians' medical rivals were not entirely unskilled in the art of using language to persuade. Despite their more knowing way with words, the physicians' sought-after dominion that seemed firmly established by century's end was hard won, and the discursive as well as practical threat to their intellectual and economic protectionism is surely implied by the frequency and vehemence of their scathing critiques. Again and again, the humanist education that enabled their eventual supremacy was invoked to assert the physicians' professional superiority over the "ignorant" surgeons and apothecaries and, especially, over those myriad irregular practitioners whose experiential epistemology challenged their own. That the physicians' discursive self-fashioning managed so long to resist the very practices they increasingly took up even as they persistently championed their own "*Art*" suggests that they were also well prepared to out-argue their professional rivals.

As much as rhetoric is "Above all," as Harley notes, "required to create new disciplines" ("Social Construction" 411), it is equally necessary to reshape the old into something new, and the physicians' eventual success at doing so is at least in part attributable to their rhetorical agility. The medical paradigm shift that began in the seventeenth century and, as well as easier access to books and publishing, is accounted for by some significant philosophical, scientific, political, and social changes was in large measure effected also by the physicians' habit of laying claim to what also served to define their opposition.[33] Thus by 1667, we meet George Castle's *The Chymical Galenist*, a work whose title alone reconciles the learned and Paracelsian, and, in 1670, *The Accomplisht Physician, the Honest Apothecary, and the Skilful Chyrurgion* attributed to physician Christopher Merrett and expressing the subtitular intention of *Detecting Their necessarry Connexion, and Dependance on each other.* Yet even those later, overt attempts at rapprochement among competing medical practices come not without the privileging and exclusionary tendencies dominant in earlier treatises. Castle's and Merrett's works may suggest that the physicians' rhetoric had become more open to medical practices once held up as insistently distinct but may have been no less contentious: we soon learn that Merrett's book also includes *Withall a Discovery of the Frauds of the Quacking Empirick, the Præscribing Surgeion,*

[33] "Since the seventeenth century," Stock notes, "the progress of medicine has relied almost entirely on biology and chemistry" (495), while Furdell argues that "the triumph of the English medical entrepreneur was due to the publication of popular books of home remedies, herbals, and wellness regimes" by which "London bookmen undermined the legal monopoly of the traditional medical establishment and assured the success of it challengers" (49). Learned medicine may have shifted its rhetorical emphases accordingly, but medical practice changed little. Throughout the eighteenth century, physicians continued to rely on Galenist theory and practices that yet focused on balancing the humours. Though, as W.R. Albury explains, "their use was now theorised in an eclectic terminology drawing from Hippocratic-Galenic humouralism, mechanical and chemical theories, and the latest results of experimental physiology and natural philosophical speculation," physicians continued to rely on the "classic therapies, such as bleeding, purging and manipulation of diet" that remained "the mainstay of medical practice in the late eighteenth century" (3).

and the Practicing Apothecary. Evidently, the volume's exposure of fraudulent practices includes those of empirics, surgeons, and apothecaries but points no accusing finger at the titular physicians who are here conspicuous in their absence, and whose College had awarded the physician–author the class of distinction some twenty years earlier.[34] Tellingly, Merrett's remains the only blameless branch of medicine.

[34] See D. E. Allen's *DNB* entry, "Merret, Christopher (1614–1695)." Cook also notes that Merrett was among a group of College Physicians interested in "the new natural philosophy, in which anatomy and physic played a major role" (*Medical Regime* 108). Though evidently interested in the "new" medicine, Merrett was loyal to the old structure the College established and upheld.

CHAPTER 3

"An Eloquent Tongue"
Physicians and Patients

Henry Peacham's 1593 *The Garden of Eloquence* invokes Horace in a dedicatory epistle reminding the reader that "in ancient time men did attribute so great opinion of wisedome to the eloquent Orators of those daies, that they called them sacred, holy, divine, & the interpreters of goddes." Next only "to the omnipotent God in the power of perswasion, by grace, & divine assistance," the quasi-divine orator is akin also to the physician, whose necessary rule as "the emperour of mens minds & affections" (Sig. A.B.iij$_v$) was also confirmed by the ancients; as James Primrose avers, "*Galen* in a peculiar book saith, that he ought to be a Philosopher; and *Hippocrates* saies, that a Physician which is a Philosopher, is God-like" (2). But it was not only physicians who invoked classical authority in asserting their right to rule. Clergyman John Dunton, whose "funeral discourses" posthumously appeared in *The House of Weeping* (1682), explicitly takes the physician's part as he advises that

> to those that come to visit us in Sickness, we are to shew a good Example of Patience and a composed Mind. And though the Disease be grievous, though many things afflict us, though some things displease us, other things are not done to our minds, never to fret and murmur. All our Troubles are to be season'd with the hope of Reward. Our Deeds and Sayings to be rendred commendable by Submission and Patience.

Urging the afflicted "to submit as well to the Physicians of the Body, as the Soul" (180), Dunton confirms the physician's authority as he advocates patient compliance.

The physician's ministrations thus also addressed "aberrations" of mind and spirit that, Lawrence Kirmayer proposes, are yet "rationalized, contained, and controlled" (325) by medicine's discursive logic.[1] Given that the Cartesian dualism to which Kirmayer's "disembodied mentality" alludes

1 Stock, on the other hand, implies that patient mentality may not have been as important in early modern medicine, given that the ancients were focused on "the body as the locus of disease" and "mind–body treatments" therefore "do not figure prominently in the writings of the founders of Western medicine, Hippocrates and Galen." Stock goes on to suggest that "this attitude was the

would only later work its full effect, the "troublesome deviance" of illness he describes (325) may have been even more difficult to accommodate in Dunton's day. Early modern physicians treated the whole patient, and they did so with the understanding, Dunton implies, that "power over passion," as Stephen Pender puts it, "is the soul of rhetoric" ("Imagination" 66). Wielding its persuasive force over an ever-reciprocal body, mind, and spirit, the physicians' rhetoric sometimes worked also to invoke the emotions that were both the cause and product of bodily illness. Particularly interested in the pathos of fear, physicians deployed its persuasive effects to professionalizing as well as patient-subduing ends. Whether warning against medical interlopers who should be fearful of dabbling in medicine, advising patients to avoid fear's plague-inducing effects, or invoking fear to effect physical cure, the physicians' collective and sometimes contradictory appeals in many ways confirm the extent of learned medicine's interest in fashioning and preserving its authority.

Yet the physicians' sometimes-extreme measures also suggest a medical authority not easily won over patients whose very need for subjection suggests an agency greater than the physicians willingly admit. As the work of medical historians from Roy Porter and Harold Cook to Monica Green and Wendy Churchill has in recent decades confirmed, patients were not always the passive consumers the physicians' rhetoric aimed to subdue. Knowledge about health and healing became more open with medicine's ongoing popularization and, as Cook points out, the "basic elements of learned medicine" were generally understood by a public aware of humoral theories as well as the Galenic "nonnaturals" of "air, diet, evacuations, exercise, sleep, and mental and emotional stimulation" over which patients had much more control (Cook, *Medical Regime* 61). As consumers, patients sometimes also held the upper hand in relationships necessarily shaped by class. In a context where education and profession in themselves had yet to confer gentility, and where those who could most afford to pay frequently out-ranked them, "physicians often had to defer to the medical wishes of their patients," Cook notes, and many "accepted or disagreed with their

distant forerunner of what has become known as the 'medical model' of illness: the view that each clinically definable condition has a single cause that can be determined, and that isolating this cause is what dictates the appropriate treatment" (494–95). The bodily focus Stock describes is, of course, a distinguishing feature of latter-day medicine. But there is no question that the humours were also thought to shape disposition and, as Freidson points out, varied definitions of illness agree that it is "a type of deviation, or deviance, from a set of norms representing health or normality." No matter its specific parameters, "in all cases" of illness, Freidson explains, "the idea of deviation from some standard" applies (207). The aim of Galenic medicine was, of course, restoring the humours to norms of ideal health.

practitioner's advice as they saw fit" (*Medical Regime* 60–61). Some early modern patients may have commanded even greater authority than those who treated them, but medical treatment cannot in any case deny the agency of subjects who alone can offer the verbal and bodily "signs" on which diagnosis and treatment depend.

Because the physicians rely on the persuasion of images, emotions, and beliefs Stephen Pender describes ("Imagination" 66), they cannot help but acknowledge the corresponding interdependence of mind, body, and spirit. Thus unable utterly to obscure the autonomy of subjects in a context where rhetoric, medicine, and religion are as symbiotic as they are separable, the physicians could neither control a discourse that was as much a part of religion as medicine, the former offering as much to empower sufferers as the latter to subdue them. As much as "medical discourses," as Margaret Healy argues, also "constitute themselves through their intersection with other discourses" (158), so are other discourses constituted by the medical. Understanding bodily affliction as a mark of divine favour, early modern sufferers also draw on the discourse of religion to discover in affliction the means of their own healing. Sometimes, as the example of John Donne that concludes this chapter suggests, the fearful and faithful found also the means to critique and thereby fashion the physicians who treated them. Strive as it might to assert dominion over diseases and patients, the language of learned medicine could not lay exclusive claim to what remains, as Foucault says, "an exegesis" harkening ever back "to the Word" (Intro.) that served patients as much as physicians.

Patients were neverthless urged to accept without question the "substantiall rules" asserted by the physican, who, according to Galen, needed also to carry "a high hand" over those "subject to miscarry" (English 13). As Edwards explains in *The Analysis of Chyrurgery*, the physician may even "refuse the cure" by withdrawing or denying care when the "disease is uncurable," the sufferer "cannot endure fit remedies," or the "cure of one disease causeth a worse." Though here upholding the precept of doing no harm, Edwards also maintains that physicians can reasonably deny treatment in cases when the "patient is disobedient, and wil not observe fit order in all things as is requisite for the cure." Invoking the *atechnic* proof of classical authority, Edwards points out that "medicine, saith Hyppocrates in his Aphorisme, was not ordained for disorderly and disobedient persons" (*Analysis* 25). Urging a top-down disregard for patients who do not properly acknowledge authority, Edwards believes that only those who respect the Galenic hierarchy mandating physicians "even as Officers over

Souldiers, and Kings over Subjects" to rule (English 15) deserve his attention and effort.[2]

Physician Thomas Chamberlayne goes beyond mere assertion to illustrate the necessity of patient subjection in *The Compleat Midwifes Practice* (1659).[3] Proving the point with the example of a woman treated by a "Chyrugeon" who beat him to the door but failed to save her, "See here how ill a thing it is to be opinionated," he concludes, "for I could easily have delivered her, if she would have been ruled by me" (17). Chamberlayne may regret the patient's unnecessary demise, but he is more bothered by patient non-compliance than harmful outcome. It is telling as well that the author of the anonymously penned *Philiatros,* a 1615 epistle *Propounded to a young Student of Physicke,* insists that it "is the duetie of the Physitian, not to forsake his Patient upon the Signes of death," yet mimics (and perhaps models) the very behaviour warned against. Abruptly abandoning the topic in the next sentence, the epistle writer claims that "occasions cut me off" and quickly moves on to a more pressing problem, the misperception that "Physicke is to easie a Studeis [sic]" and the lamentable result "that the paines of Physitians are so meanly rewarded" ("Section 13" Sig. 17_v). Dismissing the patient and turning his attention to the profession as abruptly as Chamberlayne, the *Philiatros* author also gives priority to an *exigence* evidently more urgent than correcting those who turn their backs on the dying.[4]

[2] Of course, the oft-lamented propensity for disobedience confirms that patients were quite capable of thinking and acting for themselves, and Porter is therefore right to insist that "we should stop seeing the doctor as the agent of primary care." As Porter goes on to observe, "People took care before they took physick," and "Szasz's pleas for the autonomy of the afflicted, and Goffman's studies of the Brechtian survival strategies of the inmates of total institutions, offer a salutary counterbalance, a view of lay initiative, resilience, and capacity to play the system" ("The Patient's View" 194). The physicians who assert their need for utter compliance are no doubt responding to the initiative, resilience, and agency Porter describes.

[3] Fissell notes that "because the title page lists a series of intitials, beginning with 'T.C.,'" the book is most often attributed to Chamberlayne, though "the text actually consists, in part, of translations of midwifery books by Louise Bourgeois and Jakob Rueff" ("Marketplace" 115). The mediation of women's knowledge by the men who disseminated it is discussed in Chapter 6.

[4] The *Philiatros* author points out that Sir Francis Bacon was moved also to address the physicians' self-serving habits "in his Booke of the Advancement of Learning," where he reminds the practitioner of his duty as he "urgeth" the physician to attend "his Pacient to the Death, labouring the mitigation of Paine, facilitating the passage to Death, &c." ("Section 13" Sig. C3v/17). Analyzing the rhetoric of domestic medicine in extant recipe collections, Seth Stein LeJacq notes that such works "often recorded stories of physicians and surgeons failing or abandoning their patients." As Bacon's essay confirms, evidence of patient abandonment is found in many genres; as Le Jacq explains, "These 'given over' stories are not unique to recipe books; many different sorts of people made use of them in, for instance, medical writing, advertisements and medical conflicts," their broad usefulness presenting "a strong indication of their rhetorical power" (460).

Treated as a secondary topic or as what turns out to be a mere aside in *Philiatros*, the patients whose case histories would only later become medicine's defining genre are granted little attention in texts more often intent on the self-fashioning interests of learned medicine.[5] Where patients do come up, they often shoulder the blame for bodily illnesses that bear witness to an equally deviant spirit and mind. Thomas Sherwood, who focuses also on the "Practitioner in Physick" in his 1641 *The Charitable Pestmaster, Or, the Cure of the Plague*, certainly holds sufferers blame worthy in his account of the plague's "divers causes." Echoing Browne's invoking of the Fall as an explanation for the people's misguided attraction to "popular errors," the first, Sherwood writes, "is sin, which ought to be repented of." As a "first cause" alluding to the doctrine of original sin, blame for the plague seems shared by all; at the same time, however, Sherwood's words imply individual culpability in a need for action that has only to do with the repenting believer and his maker. "The second" Sherwood identifies as "an infected and corrupted air, which should be avoided," a cause that does not hold potential sufferers accountable for the plague-bearing air, but does require that they ensure its avoidance. The third cause, "an evill diet, which should be amended," however, makes it clear that those who fail to amend by taking preventive action and therefore choose to consume what is "evill" are responsible for any ensuing infection. Sherwood's fourth and final cause, the "evill humours heaped together in the body, being apt to putrifie, and beget a Fever," does not in itself imply patient culpability; that they "must be taken away by convenient medicines" (1) does, however, place the onus on the patient to seek out the physician who is alone qualified to restore all to proper balance. Suggesting the plague sufferer's failure on four counts – to repent, to avoid infected air, to amend a poor diet, or to submit to the care of the physician whose humoral correctives would have prevented illness in the first place – Sherwood's four causes work to varying degrees to accrue blame to the sufferer. In one way or another, patient failings stand in implied and direct contrast to Galenic authority. Blaming subjects who have neither figuratively nor literally paid proper

[5] In her discussion of medical case histories, Siraisi traces their development in fifteenth-century Italy and the genre's later emergence in England. Of seventeenth-century examples, she points specifically to the work of "the Paracelsian royal physician to the early Stuarts," who accompanied the details of Issaac Casuabon's dissection with "an admiring biographical portrait and narrative of the last illness of the Calvinist scholar" ("Anatomizing the Past" 6–7). Siraisi demonstrates throughout the importance of history to physicians, including Galen, hence establishing medicine's interconnection with yet another discipline (see also Siraisi's more recent monograph, *History, Medicine, and the Traditions of Renaissance Learning* [Ann Arbor: University of Michigan Press, 2007]).

due, what claims to be a discussion of the plague proves as interested in championing those capable of treating the disease for which patients are in large measure responsible.

Where they appear at all, patients are assigned a like supporting role in most physician-authored works, not worthy of the ink shed on discrediting their many medical rivals but desirable as the foil against which the learned physician shines more brightly.[6] Dispensing advice that works equally to assert and reinforce the physician's authority, even texts offering comparatively extensive discussions of patients do not focus on their well-being so much as they deploy the afflicted to serve a rhetorical end similar to Sherwood's. Hence Boorde insists on unquestioning obedience to the "expert phisition," who alone knows "how and in what wise the body may be recovered of his infirmitie." The patient, he avers, must therefore "commit his body to the industry of his phisition" and be "at all times ready to follow" his "will, minde, and counsell." Indeed, "whosoever wil doe the contrary," Boorde insists in a spiritual appeal proved by Augustine, "doth kill himselfe that doth not observe the commandement of his physicion." According to Boorde, even the patient's household must work to "please and serve the phisition or Chirurgion honestly, and let them lack nothing, to the end, that they may be the more diligent to doe the think that they goe about: which is to recover the sicke person."[7] That Boorde deems it necessary to insist again on the physician's absolute command also points to that which threatened the physicians' enterprise: "marke this matter well," he avers, "that if there bee anye Phisition or Chirurgion, which is with anye sicke man, woman or childe, let no man disquiet them that bee in the house, nor tell them what they should doe, let everie person be tendable about them, and do as they shall command them" ("A Preamble to sicke men and to those that bee wounded" n. pag.). Whether by tending patients directly or interfering with how that tending should be done, no

[6] Lingo identifies a similar strategy in the "strong professionalizing tendency" (596) of French physicians, whose hegemonic aims included transforming healing from public spectacle to "a serious, private interaction between trained expert and submissive, loyal patient" in the medical manifestation of a larger social conflict of "insider and the outsider, elite and popular, center and margin, male and female" (597).

[7] Boorde's directive also reminds us that early modern households were often well populated and complex. Though we may now "tend to think of sickness and the other great bodily events as quintessentially individual, private experiences," such thinking, as Porter points out, "would be a mistake for communities in the past." Despite the involvement of one's relatives and even community in the history of suffering, however, "the story of family medicine," Porter remarks, "remains curiously neglected" ("The Patient's View" 194).

competing domestic healer is to challenge the physician's preeminence or question his command.[8]

Persuading patients to obey and other healers to acquiesce demands that, in addition to Grammar and Logic, Boorde's physician need also "have a rethorick or an eloquent tongue, the which should bee placable to the hearers of his words" ("The Preface" n. pag.).[9] Urging compliance, Boorde's appeal to pathos aims to strike fear as he forthrightly declares his purpose to "advertise everye man and woman, of what degree of estate soever they be, lacking the speculation of phisick, to beware to minister mediciens." No matter what level of education, practical training, or self-knowledge any man or woman might command, it is always dangerous to do so, he insists, "if they have not a doctours learning." Boorde argues that such meddlers may not only "doe great harme" of the bodily kind but will "for their presumption" also "offend both God and man." Implying that medical interlopers may even risk damage to their immortal souls, Boorde appeals also to the spirit in invoking the greatest fear of all ("The Preface" n. pag.). Aiming to ensure a "placable" patient, Boorde's rhetoric points to an *exigence* nowhere more urgent than in his two-fold appeal to the persuasion of fear.

Addressing and sometimes inculcating the illness-inspired trepidation inevitable in an age of high mortality, the rhetoric of learned medicine frequently relied on appeals that, as Beth Innocenti puts it, "are designed

[8] Household healers may have presented an even greater threat to the physicians' hegemony than their professional rivals, given that "empiric medicine," as Wear explains, "was analogous to the centuries-old practice of offering remedies to family and friends" that "were sometimes equated with empirical medicine," and the physicians were "seen as attacking both" ("Continuity" 309). Curtailing the participation of others is not, however, the aim of all physicians. Stephen Bradwell, a London physician motivated by his love for the city, published his *Physick for the Sickness, Commonly called the Plague* with the subtitular aim of acquainting the reader "With all the Particular Signes and Symptoms, whereof the most are too ignorant." Bradwell is thus willing to share knowledge and practice: "The information within," the title page also proclaims, is "collected, Out of the Choycest Authors, and Confirmed with good Experience; for the benefit and Preservation of all, both Rich and Poore."

[9] As demonstrated in the preceding chapters, rhetoric was important to physicians in delineating and preserving the bounds of their profession. Yet effective rhetoric, Nicholas Fonteyn writes in *The Womans Doctour* (1652), is crucial also to the effectiveness of physicians who write about healing. "Modern men," he notes, "also have been stirred up to their [women's] defence, as Mercurialis, and Mercatus," but they have done so with varying degrees of success: "the former indeed with sufficient elegance, but the latter with so much tediousness, and confusion; that you may sooner finde your Patient dead, then a remedy in his writings for her recovery." Using language well, according to Fonteyn, can be a matter of life and death, and the bookish physicians are sometimes not suited to the challenge. In an attempt "to correct this inconvenience," he goes on to observe, a certain "Rodericus a Castro engaged his pen in their quarrell, but with no great successe" because "his writings are more learned, then usefull" (The First book of womens diseases, "The Proem by the Author" Sig. A2v).

to induce action – to generate persuasive force for addressees to act in order to avoid a fearful outcome" (273). Like the rhetors challenged by those who, Thomas Hobbes argues, "*fear* little" because "they have suffered already," the physicians also worked hard to put "put *Fear* into the Auditor" (56). Using like means to justify a curative end that admitted no qualms about their often-shameless fear mongering, they sometimes aimed to instill the fear of fear itself. Discoursing at length about fear's dangers in his 1636 *Physick for the Sickness, Commonly called the Plague,* Stephen Bradwell maintains: "I need bring no Examples for proofe: for in every place I heare living witnesses of such as dyed of the Plague, stricken onely with the fear of it: And therefor I cannot think any mans ignorance can plead against it" (37). According to Bradwell, fear impedes healing in both bringing on disease and preventing effective treatment and is invoked in an *entechnic* appeal to pathos so persuasive it requires "no Examples for proofe."

Fear is thought also to inhibit the efficacy of treatment. Itemizing what is "required at the present time of bleeding," Edwards advises that the ministering "Artist" needs to have the physical advantages of "cleare and perfect" light and sight as well as the intellect to consider thoughtfully the "best way" to proceed among three kinds of incisions. The patient, however, needs "three things" that require not intellectual discernment but the application of will and control over passion. Submitting to the act of bleeding, Edwards notes, demands the patient's "quietnesse" of body and mind, "willing obedience," and a constitution "bold and stout of courage" and "voyd of feare" (*Analysis* Sig. $G3_r$/45). Like Bradwell, Edwards seems to advocate the practitioner's appeal to a pathos that, in invoking courage and discouraging fear, may serve more to enable than constrain the patient–subject. At the same time, however, their warnings against fear work in tandem with their self-fashioning priorities. In Edwards's case, the practitioner's status as an "Artist" alone asserts his authority and, in Bradwell's, the expressed need to "bring no Examples for proofe" confirms an ethos whose superiority is so readily apparent he need not even bother with the usual kinds of evidence – only "ignorance," Bradwell maintains, would deny the veracity of what he need only assert.

The physicians sometimes advocate fear as an emotion to be invoked instead of avoided. In his 1656 *The Doctresse,* for instance, Richard Bunworth ends his chapter of recommendations "for the falling down of the Womb" with what he claims to be a tried-and-true cure. "Able Physitians," he advises, "report that some women have been cured of this distemper by fear onely." As it turns out, Bunworth's cure for the errant womb depends on the physician's rhetorical skill. "Let the Patient be perswaded," he advises, "that the bearing down or swelling must be seared with a hot iron." Relying on the visual as well as the verbal, the persuasive force of the latter is supplemented by a gruesome ritual performed before the patient's eyes: "let an iron be put into the fire," Bunworth recommends, "and other such like preparations made in the sight of the Patient." Doing so "that she may really think that she must be immediately cauterized" will effect cure, he maintains, as "the apprehension and fear of this will, without doubt, cause the Womb to shrink up, and return to its proper place" (37). Treating the ailing body through the force of a fearful spirit, Bunworth's cure offers an extreme but telling illustration of the emotion's persuasive necessity.

Whether evoked, prohibited, or prescribed, fear works to fashion an early modern patient susceptible to a variety of rhetorical manipulations, both verbal and visual, whose collective contradictions would presumably go unnoticed. Taken together, the varied and inconsistent uses of fear seen in Boorde, Bradwell, Edwards, and Bunworth suggest that successful recovery depended not on the subjects' ability to reason against the physicians' arguments or to participate in the physical process of healing, but on compliance, passivity, and acquiescence.[10] But we cannot, as Michael Stolberg reminds us, "rely on the often one-sided polemical accounts of learned physicians" in the face of other evidence to suggest that even "less-educated patients also met with medical professionals eye to eye" (75).[11] As manipulative as their various appeals may sometimes seem, the physicians' coercion suggests even in its tyranny a rhetoric whose persuasive success depended to some extent on recruiting and thereby acknowledging the active, inner life of the patient. Though aiming explicitly to encourage compliance, such agency is implicit in the patient's recognized ability to infer and imagine the uterine cauterization Bunworth's charade implies

10 From the physician's perspective, the early modern patient may not differ significantly from more recent constructions: "All too often," Garden laments in her study of patient involvement in the healing process, "the person who is chronically ill or disabled is reduced to a stock role as a pitiable figure who serves to affirm others' normalcy and well-being, or as the 'good patient,' who must bear up stoically under the weight of suffering" ("Narrative" 122). The physicians' rhetoric thus shapes through inculcated submission the "pitiable figure" and the "good patient" subject to the many fear-centred appeals to pathos as well as the physician's understood authority.

11 Chagrined by the healing efforts of their competition the learned physicians may have been, but their relationship with their sick subjects may also be characterized by the "complex mix of confidence and distrust" Stolberg observes (71). It may also be that, as Stolberg argues, "patients of the time tended to be in a significantly stronger position than they are today" (75), and the physicians' intently subjugating rhetoric therefore aimed by overcompensation to remediate a lesser power differential.

and the imaginative potential acknowledged in Bradwell's expressed belief that some have "dyed of the Plague, stricken onely with the fear of it."

Bradwell goes on to recognize more directly the patient's independence of mind and spirit as he further validates his caveat against fear. "Yet I will give a reason for it," he explains, "because of all Passions, *Feare* is the most pestilently pernicious; *And this it is*: Feare enforces the vitall Spirits to retire inward to the heart: By which retyring they leave the outward parts infirme, as appeares plainly by the palenesse and trembling of one in great feare." In a telling instance of the *enargeia* that is a virtue of effective style, Bradwell suggests a measure of patient agency as he brings before the eyes images of war aiming to render visible the doleful effects of fear: "So that the walls being forsaken (which are continually besieged by the outward ayre) in comes the enemy boldly; the best spirits that should expelled them having cowardly sounded retreat" (37). Though retreating "cowardly" in the face of invading illness, those "best spirits" also imply the potential to resist, to expel fear with a bold and best spirit. Invoking an analogy of evaporation, Bradwell moves from the vividness of armed conflict to the discourse of natural philosophy in describing fearful effects that "draw in with them such evill vapours as hang about the outward pores" as he alludes to the spirit with an adjectival "evill" linked also to the body. Offering a more concrete simile whose equivalence is found in the way "the Sunne drawes toward it the vapours of the Earth," Bradwell concludes in *enthymematic* appeal to reason over emotion, the unstated premise of which affirms the reciprocity of body and spirit. "And hence is it," he infers, "that *Feare* brings *Infection* sooner then any other occasion" (37). Bradwell's account of a fear he also claims "dissolves the Brayne" (35) figures a mind yet to be disembodied. In doing so, he alludes also to the tandem understanding that, as Stock observes, "at the beginning of the modern period, mind–body practices were mainly found in the ill-defined territory between magic, medicine, and religion" (495). Like the products of magic, Bradwell's ephemeral vapours are understood not in the particulars of their composition or the means of their working, but in their evident, memorable, and equal effect on mind, body, and spirit.

Bringing before the eyes fear's visible effects, Bradwell's imagery functions also as the kind of "rhetorical therapy" Stephen Pender describes as treatment reliant on "rhetoric's ability to make the absent present" and "to insinuate rather than baldly, logically argue" as the physicians profess to do. Bradwell's formulation in some ways takes the form of argument, especially in a concluding statement confirming the role of fear in bringing about infection, yet its persuasive force is the product of insinuation achieved through rhetoric's "ability to make the absent present" in a vivid and largely metaphorical accounting of fear's effects. As Pender also notes, "it was commonplace for ancient and early modern rhetoricians to associate vivid description with the arousal of emotion," and the physicians' multiple uses of fear to ends at one with the rhetorician's attest to an understanding that permeates all aspects of early modern medicine, that is, the belief that "the mind is moved by emotion, and that movement is dependent on images." In many ways, the physicians' rhetoric proceeds from the premise Pender descibes, that "only when we are moved and conceive images of things do we adapt ourselves to, and understand, a speech or a situation, a conversation or an event" ("Imagination" 66). In their discursive treatment of patients, then, the physicians at least imply that "it takes two to make a medical encounter" ("The Patient's View" 175), as Porter would have it, and they may appeal to imagery as much to encourage inward change as to force outward compliance.

In his strikingly titled 1640 guidebook, *The Marrow of Physicke: Or, A learned Discourse of the severall parts of mans Body*, Thomas Brugis speaks of emotional effects more literally than metaphorically. Addressing the psyche and the emotions that go with it, Brugis's preface takes up the "Perturbations or passions of the mind" that include suffering "either by joy, hope, love, hatred, anger, and the like." The mind does not, however, suffer alone, and Brugis makes clear that such emotions also "bring great mutations in the body." The effects of mind on body are "most necessary to be remarked," he insists, "because of the great chances that ensue thereupon." Though the extent of physical damage done "by these motions" can vary, given that "the heate and spirits are sometimes gently, sometimes violently diffused over all the body," and can even facilitate the "enjoying of the present or future good," the "spirits" he describes can also do much harm. Some patients adversely affected by spirits invoked by the imaginative mind have evidently suffered the worst damage of all: "by receiving any affront," Brugis writes, "many have so exceedingly been moved, that they have died" (Sig. $K3_v$/70).

Brugis's more direct approach may also signal a keener awareness of the importance of rhetorical choices to his self-fashioning, an understanding he confirms also by disclaimer. Addressing the "Gentle Reader," he claims for "a principall aime at my countries good" in publishing his receipts, making clear that he does so with no desire "to set forth an eloquent and lofty stile (as it were some fancy delighting history) but a plaine way to helpe the poorer sort." Hence, he goes on, "I here produce a thing serious, and for the generall good." Following Cicero's civic injunction not to pay primary "regard to our owne particular profit," which for Brugis would mean "keeping the secrets of Physick so close" as they have been, he advocates and models a discourse more open than distinctive. Apart from the obvious exclusion of the unlettered, Brugis avoids the protectionist bent characteristic of the physicians' rhetoric more generally. Refusing to exclude by means of lofty style, esoteric terminology, or archaic language, Brugis writes in a way inclusive of those who might otherwise "perish for want of meanes to procure the advise of a physician" and who, "perhaps with a little instructions [sic], they might have cured themselves" ("The Preface to the Reader" n. pag.). Whether dispensing rhetorically appropriate "instructions," as does Brugis, or advocating therapies that are deeply and inevitably rhetorical, as do Bunworth, Boorde, Edwards, and Bradwell, the physicians prove equally aware of language's capacity to heal.

Like the rhetoricians as well, the physicians understood the importance of not only genesis but also analysis to their enterprise, and diagnoses had long been inferred and treatments devised by listening to and interpreting signs offered both verbally and visually.[12] The necessity of "reading" their patients English's translation of *Galen's Method* makes clear. Acknowledging that "every nature doth not require alike remedies," the text advocates the adaptive approach necessitated by humoural theory: thus "the more weak and tender" a nature is, "the more gentle should the medicaments be," while "the stronger and dryer the nature is, the stronger should be the medicaments." To discover where effective treatment may fall on the continuum of strong and weak, "the nature of the Patient is the first thing to be considered" (Sig. C_r/49), and the physician need therefore "admit a latitude to the Patient" who may know more of "some contingent and accidentall things which the Nicety of his constitution doth require." As much as medical writers might insist that the physician encompasses "all things materiall and substantiall in medicine," familiarity with the particulars of their own constitutions grants patients a further measure of agency,

12 Discussing diagnosis and narrative, Lee T. Pearcy points out, "Although Hippocratic medicine understood the utility of listing symptoms, and later medicine exploited logical and rhetorical schemes of classification and division, ancient physicians from the Hippocratics until late antiquity retained the habit of describing disease as a story," thus describing a narrative mode focused on diseases rather than patients. Drawing the inevitable connection of medicine to rhetoric, however, he goes on to note that "physiological concepts articulate and shape their stories, just as rhetorical divisions and narrative patterns inform nonmedical narrations." Even unpopulated narratives of disease share the moments of climax and denouement of any good story, he argues, for "crisis days are expected stations in the tale of an illness, and the Galenic schema protopathy-sympathy-idiopathy constitutes a form in which to narrate the dynamic course of a disease from beginning through middle to end" (601).

and English thus excludes from the physician's purview the non-naturals that include "niceties and various contingences of the Patients disposition, dyet and such like" ("Comment" 13).

Even texts not dominated by Galenic theory admit a degree of patient agency, for successful diagnosis and treatment also depended on knowledge accessible only through patients. Bradwell's treatise on the plague thus advises "the way to know this *Sickness* from all others" he has "found out (by certain Signes)." Though Bradwell acknowledges, "It will not be amisse out of learned Authoritie to teach you how to know, whether a man at the first taking or soone after, be likely to be recovered or no," in the case of plague, the physician would do better to read and interpret what is proffered rather than consult "learned Authoritie."[13] "If one be taken with the first Signes of *Sinking of his Spirits, causelesse Sadnesse, shortnesse of Breath* on the suddaine, that hee cannot forbeare *Sighing*," he writes, "yet knowes no cause why" (50), then the patient presents visible, accessible signs of one suffering from plague. Those signs do not, however, tell the whole story. Plague's indicators may be physically manifest in sunken spirits, baseless sorrow, and short breath, but the diagnosis is finally determined only with confirmation by elimination, that the patient "knowes no cause why" (50).

That patients have a semiotic and collaborative role to play in diagnosis as well as recovery is confimed in "recent years," John L. Coulehan notes, in which "a number of writers have proposed that we add *patient as text, doctor as interpreter* to the set of metaphors that we use to describe the physician–patient relationship" (116).[14] Bradwell's early modern reading of

[13] As Harley notes, "The Galenic or Enlightenment physician's diagnosis depended upon an interpretation of signs and story which drew upon natural philosophy and medical theory." Signs did not, however, operate out of context, and the physicians also "incorporated judgements concerning the moral and social standing of the patient" ("Social Construction" 420).

[14] Shifting focus to "the interpretive function of clinical medicine," Coulehan suggests, promises greater insight into the nature of "physician–patient encounters" (116). The interpretive role of later-day physicians set out in the work of Good and Delvecchio-Good and described by Coulehan as the two premises of their "cultural hermeneutic model" proceeds from the premise that "all realities of illness are fundamentally semantic" to the extent that "they are constructed from, and experienced within, the sick person's world of symbols, the network of meanings through which he or she understands 'reality.'" Hence all encounters between afflicted and healer become "fundamentally hermeneutic or interpretive" to the extent that "interpreting and translating the patient's experience are a central feature of medicine" (112). Coulehan's case studies focus on three points of interdependent connection, the empathic, narrative, and cultural. The first requires "listening to and 'being with' an ill person," the second arises from the first "when stories told by patient and physician 'fit' together," the third from the second "when an illness has strong cultural meaning and the physician is able to provide a culturally accepted remedy for the patient's suffering" (113). The process Coulehan describes is not new, however. Even Petrarch recognized medicine's "absolute need for interpretation," pointing in his "Invectives against the Doctor" to the difficulty of reading the "mute signs" interpreted through a "medical semiotic" whose treatments, Streuver argues, depended on neither "words" nor "colors" but equally mute drugs (662).

patient signs describes a similarly hermeneutic approach, one that depends not on the fixed meaning of physical signs per se, but on those signs as they are described by the patient and subsequently interpreted by the physician. Contrary to what we might expect from a text predicated on the teachings of Galen and Hippocrates, Bradwell offers an interpretive model that does not proceed from abstract theories of the disease to its manifestation in an individual, but moves from particular symptoms to diagnosis. Positing a more explicitly inductive hermeneutic for treating "the immoderate flowing of the Courses," the anonymously translated *The Compleat Doctoress* (1656) recommends finding "the signes by conversing with, and questioning the sick woman." Granting a measure of control to the female patient, however, the story she writes is one with which "you may easily make your selfe acquainted" (25). Thus alluding to some deeply entrenched notions about the sex so often construed as dangerously loquacious while implying an opportunity for some self-fashioning of their own, the hermeneutic model advocated here seems to take with one hand what it gives with the other. Supported by evidence reaching all the way back to the Fall, the discursive echoes of the many and oft-repeated injunctions against female speech proved with the damage done by a disobedient, deteminedly self-fashioning Eve resound even in assurances of easy access to the text necessary for proper diagnosis.

Alluding to some scripturally supported notions about women, regularly invoking the textual authority of learned medicine, quoting "the Poet" Ovid's epigram "The Doctour cannot still successefull be, / Sometimes the evill gets the victory" (Sig. $C2_v$) in both Latin and English, and appending the work of "Nicholas Fontanus" in the *Of Womens Diseases* comprising its "Second Book," *The Compleat Doctoress* is everywhere marked by its author's (or compiler's) immersion in a deeply textual and intertextual tradition.[15] There is no denying that medical discourses "constitute themselves through their intersection with other discourses" (Healy 158), and that all

[15] *The Compleat Doctoress* argues that "womens diseases are divided into foure Classes, whereof the first containeth the diseases that are common to all women: the second comprehendeth such as are peculiar to Widowes, and Virgins; The third specifieth those Affects that concern barren women, and such as are fruitfull; And the fourth treateth of such disease, as befall Women with Childe, and Nurses" (3), and in doing so evinces an awareness of categories as gendered as they are medical. Presenting theories and practices centred on a woman's "Courses" and accounting anomalies to one or another problem with the humours, the book is also sharply focused on Galen and includes the requisite deference to Hippocrates and Artistotle. Aimed at a general audience, however, *The Compleat Doctoress* claims on its frontispiece to have been "faithfully translated out of Latine into English for a common good," and that it is also "Safe in the Composition," "Pleasant in the Use," and "Effectual in the Operation." The "Second Book," *Of Womens Diseases*, is a reprinting of Nicholas Fonteyn's *The Womans Doctor*.

interpreters of illness-related "texts" also "engage," as Stock puts it, "in quasi-literary studies of the dramas, narratives, and rituals that take place during the healing process" (494).[16] Such a "meaning-centered model" of medical practice, as Coulehan calls it, has come to the forefront of much research into medicine as it was practised in the past as well as currently, and it is one that connects in important ways with Porter's insistence on a revisionist history that includes the patient's perspective. Though early modern practitioners are not often explicit in acknowledging their role as interpreters of patient narratives in a body of work notably bereft of patient stories, treatises like Bradwell's and *The Compleat Doctoress* suggest an interdependence many are unwilling expressly to admit.[17]

Patients may be inculcated to the habit of obedience, but the physicians' complaints about unruly patients equally imply that submission is always by choice. The patient is thus akin to the faithful believer, whose doctrinal obedience "unexercised and unbreathed" not only would qualify as the kind of "excremental whiteness" (10) Milton famously derides in *Areopagitica*, but would also be impossible without the free will that remains even for one grievously curtailed by fear. In this as well, the discourse of medicine is akin to the rhetoric of religion, where fear is a familiar Judeo-Christian trope. Appealing to a pathos enabled by the Christian reader's fear of God, John Prideaux's 1659 publication on "sacred eloquence" confirms that divine language is not always kind. "*The word of God*," he notes in reference to Hebrews, "*is quick and powerfull, and sharper then any two-edged sword, piercing even to the dividing asunder of soul and spirit, and of the joints and marrow, and is a discerner of the thoughts and intents of the beast, Heb.* 4. 12" (Sig. A2$_r$/2). Uniting the physical "joints and marrow" with the metaphysical "soul and spirit," Prideaux's imagery figures a divine utterance afflicting body and soul. The religious writer Thomas Calvert instead offers a metaphor of written language in his curative *Heartsalve for a Wounded Soule* (1647): "We do not always finde God writing pleasant Epistles to his

[16] Doing so comes with a caveat, however. As Garden points out in her discussion of empathy, "just as imagining the patient's perspective can diminish the patient's authority rather than provide insight, studying literature as a means of mediating the overwhelming impact of suffering can distract physicians and trainees from real suffering" ("Empathy" 563–64). Considering the patient's perspective in abstracted form, in other words, threatens empathy by turning attention toward the effects of represented suffering on readers and away from the actual affliction and its consequences.

[17] Churchill's study concludes that early modern female patients "may not have been entirely autonomous consumers" but were not utterly subordinate either. Especially those "who belonged to the upper sectors of society" and those of all classes "who presented ailments invoving female-specific anatomy," women were "capable of expressing agency when it came to making medical decisions about their bodies" (225).

children," he notes, but "sometimes writes bitter things" (68). In religious discourse, however, fear and affliction work not only destructively.[18]

In her seminal work *The Body in Pain*, Elaine Scarry points to the seemingly endless scenes of divinely imposed injuries found in the Hebrew Bible: "they recur so frequently," she observes,

> that no reader, Jewish or Christian, will have failed to notice them, and few readers, Jewish or Christian, will have failed to be troubled by them. God's invisible presence is asserted, made visible, in the perceivable alterations he brings about in the human body: in the necessity of human labor and the pains of child birth, in a flood that drowns, in a plague that descends on a house, in the brimstone and fire falling down on a city … and so on, on and on. (183)

For the Hebrew God, the power to afflict is as important as the power to heal, and both are integrally bound up with the Word. Their parallel presentation in a highly rhetorical passage from Deuteronomy underscores the centrality of language in every divine act: "See now that I, even I, am he, and there is no god with me: I kill, and I make alive; I wound, and I heal: neither is there any that can deliver out of my hand" (32.39). The ending *antistrophe* of repeated words that end the two opening clauses ("that I, even I"), together with the *anaphora* that begins the subsequent four, mimics the alpha-to-omega omniscience and omnipotence of the divine "I," thus illustrating the oneness of God and His Word. The passage also presents the *hypozeuxis* of varied repetition (the "I" remains the same, but the verb changes), the *asyndeton* of punctuation without conjunction, and the *isocolon* of clausal balance, which together enact the endless (and perhaps inevitable) cycle of wounding and healing, death and resurrection set in motion by the Word.

The passage from Deuteronomy thus formally replicates the larger scriptural pattern Scarry identifies. Writing that "man can only be created once, but once created, he can be endlessly modified; wounding re-enacts the creation because it re-enacts the power of alteration that has its first profound occurrence in creation" (183), Scarry also reiterates a cycle of creation and re-creation that was a given in the early modern narrative of devotion. Rather than the locus of complaint, however, divinely ordained suffering was more often met with the discourse of patient tolerance shared by medicine. The decorous response was not "to murmure

[18] To the extent that it plays a role in generating the Word, God's unkindness may also create. In his rhetorical analysis of Paul's epistle to the Philippians, Gregory Bloomquist suggests as much in showing that suffering may also be "a crucial mechanism in the birth and growth of the gospel" (277).

against the dispensations of God," as Samuel Clarke advises in his 1659 *Marrow of Divinity*, but to "shew Christian fortitude notwithstanding, and overcoming all these assaults" (56). Echoing the recommendations of physicians like Boorde, writers both secular and religious urge acceptance, and even alacrity, in the face of endless suffering. Conflating divine wounder and healer, "neither *rage* at the *Chirurgion*, as mad-men," Richard Younge recommends in his 1654 *A Sovereign Antidote against All Grief* as he urges the afflicted not to "swoun under his hand, as *Milk-sops*; but consider with whom thou hast to do: *The Lord, the Lord strong, merciful, and gracious, slow to anger, and abundant in goodness and truth*" (165).

Though accessible only in partnership with the faith necessary to trust even in the possibility of healing, wounds both physical and spiritual may be what give "sacred eloquence" form in the first place; that Scriptural *enargeia* seems so often to depend on physical suffering inflicted by a God whose Logos is also the ultimate healer may in itself suggest as much. The therapeutic logos integral to Hippocratic medicine, the "reason" and "word" Pedro Laín Entralgo once described as encompassing "question, prescription, instrument of prestige, means of enlightenment, and persuasive agent" (152), was equally important to the Judeo-Christian tradition and most familiar, perhaps, as the Psalmist's divine physician who "healeth the broken in heart, and bindeth up their wounds" (Ps. 147.3). As early modern writers are wont to do with all things biblical, they invoke the metaphor tirelessly, and God the healer appears in countless early modern treatises. In his 1649 *Cause and Cure of a Wounded Conscience*, for example, Thomas Fuller responds to the rhetorical question of Proverbs 18.14, "But a wounded conscience who can bear," with the metaphorically fitting answer, "God, like a wise Surgeon, would not open that wound which he never intended to cure" (6), while Younge's explicitly curative treatise calls God "the All-wise *Physician*" who knows that mortification is often "the fittest *medicine* for our souls *sickness*, and that we cannot otherwise be *cured*" (165).

The religious intersects with the medical even in the discourse of the rhetorically despotic Boorde, who recognizes the reciprocity of body and spirit, and insists on patient acquiescence only after asserting the necessity of devotion. The mark of that devotion is, of course, patient emulation of Christ's suffering. The necessary fortitude Boorde writes so adamantly about comes, he says, only when the patient is able "to fire his heart and minde in Christs death and passion, and to call to his remembrance, what paine, what adversitie, what penurie, and povertie Christ did sufrer for us" (Sig. Aiiii$_r$). Accordingly, Boorde avers that patients must focus not on their own desires or exercise their own agency, but advises that "every sicke man, & all other men the which have any infirmitie, sicknes, or impediment" must instead "above all thinges to pacifie himselfe, or to arme himselfe with patience" as he concentrates not on his illness but, like a good Christian, transcends his bodily suffering to await and accept whatever may come ("A Preamble to sicke men and to those that bee wounded" n. pag.). Patients may not assume discernibly active roles in healing, but Boorde makes clear that recovery nevertheless depends on the ability of the afflicted effectively "to pacifie himself."[19] The opportunity and state of mind prerequisite to doing so may be among the "Advantages of Sicknesse" Jeremy Taylor writes of in his 1651 *Rule and Exercise of Holy Dying*. Illness, as he puts it, is "a little image of the state of blessed Souls, or of Adams early morning in Paradise, free from the troubles of lust, and violencies of anger, and the intricacies of ambition, or the restlesnesse of covetousnesse." Forcing an inward turn, affliction can occasion spiritual growth, providing the place where "his soul shall finde some rest from labouring in the galleys, and baser captivity of sin" (109). As Taylor's words indicate, opportunity is found also in obedient acceptance; the possibility of recovery therefore depends to some extent on patient participation that cannot be utterly divorced from the rhetorical and practical application of healing.

Both Boorde's and Taylor's formulations of how patients might respond to illness actively and advantageously thus confirm something of "the dynamic interplay between sufferers and practitioners that," Porter argues, "requires study." The potential for such "dynamic interplay" is at least implied by the fruitful suffering Boorde and Taylor find in the willing submission of a subject who is not static, an implication further suggesting the advantages of Porter's bottom-up approach, offering as it does a reinflected perspective that may do more to "put medical history back on its feet" than one that for too long focused first and primarily on the physician. Hence it seems clear that beginning with physicians may indeed lend greater credence to the authority they were also determined to uphold, reinforcing in the process the hegemony claimed by learned medicine in the longstanding "tug-of-war" of "supply and demand, patient power and doctor power" Porter describes ("The Patient's View" 185). Yet, as much as the physicians' texts depict an interplay between sufferers and caregivers

[19] Early modern urgings toward mindfulness suggest that Stock may thus overstate his point when he suggests that "it is not to earlier medical practices that we should look in order to find predecessors for contemporary applications" of mind to matter, but he does not completely miss the mark in suggesting that we need also (though perhaps not primarily) to look "to the history of meditation itself" (497).

aiming to assign all healing power to the latter, and as much as learned medicine's hegemonic enterprise may have succeeded in focusing our attention on the physician and his profession, the early modern patient is not without a voice or the potential, however latent, to respond unironically to the proverbial and metaphorical injunction to "heal thyself" (Luke 4:23) anticipated by Christ in mockery of his return to Nazareth. Because it accrues not only in conjunction with but in much the same way as the spiritual kind, the "patient power" Porter insists upon cannot be utterly occluded or even denied in early modern medical thinking.

Addressing the ill directly in "A Preamble to sicke men and to those that bee wounded," Boorde even advises patients to draw on that power, arguing that patience and fortitude will do much to "Mittigate his paines & anguish." Urging as well the habits inherited from the Christian meditative tradition, Boorde confirms the correspondence of body and spirit in advocating a program of recovery that depends on imagining the suffering of another as much as Bunworth's cauterizing charade depends for its curative force on the imagined suffering of oneself. Hence it is necessary that "every sicke person stick as fast to Christ in his paynes and sicknes" as, Boorde adds in the proportional drawing of a memorable and visceral analogy aimed imaginatively to unite the suffering of the patient and that of the Saviour who "did sticke fast to the Crosse." Only once the afflicted person has deployed the imagination in service of soul, Boorde says, "then let the patient provide for his body" (Sig. Aiiii$_r$). Imaginatively invoking Christianity's most meaningful sign, "medicine and religion emerge as parallel semiotic endeavors" in a prescription of crucifixion enabled by the ability to deploy "canons of wisdom and careful observation to derive meaning in suffering" (699) in a way akin to that Jacalyn Duffin points to in her study of canonization and miracles. That body and spirit were integrally bound up in early modern healing practices – and thus necessarily dependent also on the contributions of patients whose salvation demanded the active virtue espoused so adamantly by protestant and puritan theology – may be most salient in those moments when the discouses of religion and medicine explicitly converge.

Perhaps nowhere do rhetoric, medicine, and religion more famously meet than in John Donne's 1624 illness-inspired meditations collectively known as *Devotions upon Emergent Occasions*.[20] Given that Donne was an

[20] George Herbert wrote from a patient's perspective as well, and his various lyrics on illness may be among his most familiar. A number of critics have considered Donne's and Herbert's poems in relation to one another and, tellingly perhaps, have paid particular attention to how the illness-inspired writing of these two ordained priests in the English church function as appeals to the

ordained priest and not a physician, it comes as no surprise that his own discourse of illness and healing is more closely aligned with the physician–clerics' than that of learned medicine, though the *Devotions* also negotiates and on occasion replicates some of what shapes and defines the latter.[21] Without learned medicine's professionalizing agenda, however, Donne is more willing to recognize the paradox expressed in Greene's two-sided coin of "Humanist pride and humanist despair" (9). Ever the despairing humanist yet knowing rhetor, "Oh miserable abundance, O beggarly riches!" Donne laments in the antithetical *exclamatio* of his fourth meditation. As the *exergasia* that "repeats the same thought in many figures" (Lanham 74) and leads to the consequently amplified but unanswerable *erotema*, the figure underscores the problem of medicine's profound ignorance: "how much," Donne asks rhetorically, "doe wee lacke of having *remedies* for everie disease, when as yet we have not *names* for them?" (9).

Questioning the limits of learned medicine while seeking "a literary form suitable for the expression of what was an almost ineffable experience" (29), as Thomas J. Morrissey puts it, Donne quickly offers up a provisional answer of humanist pride. Valorized as the "*Hercules* against these *Gyants*, these *Monsters*;" Donne fashions a physician who "musters up al the forces of the other world, to succour this" and is akin to that of the overreaching Hart as he calls on "all Nature to relieve Man." Championing the learned practitioner's rightful dominion, Donne advises us also to remember that "we *are not* the *Phisician*," and "heere we shrinke in our proportion, who are *Phisicians* to themselves." Unlike the hart or the dog who knows to ingest certain herbs or grass to expel arrows and poison, "man hath not that *innate instinct*, to apply these naturall medicines to his present danger, as those inferiour creatures have; he is not his owne *Apothecary*, his owne

divine. That the devotional is never far from early modern thinking, and is integrally connected with rhetoric and medicine, Narveson makes clear in a discussion of perceptions and representations of the body in Stuart England that includes Donne. From the example of "Herbert's varied attitudes toward food," however, she argues that those expressed are also "articulations of multiple discourses available to early modern believers to address the multiple perspectives from which the problem of corporeality presented itself." Even the variances seen in Herbert's work, she posits, cannot deny that "these discourses were so firmly established in the devotional tradition that a person could employ one or another in turn, or even in fruitful cross-fertilization," so internalized in early modern thinking and discourse, "the gaps or contradictions between them passing unnoticed, each one delineating the structure of the self from its own perspective" (332–33). Narveson would surely agree that the point she makes applies also to Donne.

21 Though Donne's *Devotions* is frequently scrutinized as an early modern account of illness, there has been little discussion of how his rhetoric reflects and sometimes enacts the medical-professional debate even as it serves to represent and cope with bodily illness. Clara Lander and Jonathan Goldberg made their contributions in 1971, while Stephen Pender's 2003 article considers the *Devotions* in light of early modern medical thought rather than its author's personal views on illness.

Phisician, as they are" ("Meditation IV" 9). Though Donne here may also despair of medicine's potential to do any good without the understanding granted to other creatures but not humanity, he is more intent on asserting that those who are not physicians should not presume their function, and his dismissal of the potential to use and understand "naturall medicines" at least alludes to an empirical species of healing whose practical orientation seems misguided at best and dangerous at worst.[22]

Taking the physician's part over several early meditations, the *Devotions* turns its primary focus to an author equally intent on asserting agency. Given that, as Nancy Selleck explains, "some humoral treatises seem to aim specifically at increasing their readers' sense of autonomy, offering greater knowledge and control of their own humoral makeup as a means of self-fashioning" (153), Galenic healing was especially receptive to encompassing the emotional and spiritual world of the patient even as it insisted on the physician's overriding expertise. Hence the patient Donne's self-fashioning reveals a correspondingly greater reliance on the emotional appeal of pathos than the ethos so important to the learned physicians' self-fashioning. As Selleck also notes, "humoral medicine is both psychology and physiology" (152), and there is little doubt that Donne's meditations offer a means of expressing, exploring, and coping with a life-altering illness that afflicts psychologically as well as physically.[23] It is the focus on mind and spirit that ultimately distinguishes the professionalizing rhetoric of the physician–clerics from that of their medical competition, an emphasis evident also in the devotional orientation of an illness narrative that does not, and perhaps cannot, uphold without compromise the distinctions the learned physicians paradoxically insist upon. For Donne, rhetoric, religion, and medicine are not forced into uneasy separation but are explicitly interconnected and ever interdependent.

Though taking illness as its topic, the *Devotions* may be first and foremost, as Stephen Pender claims, "a spiritual autobiography" ("Essaying

[22] Referring to Donne's satire "Away thou fondling motley humourist," Selleck points to how its use of " 'Galenists' and 'chemics' invokes the competition between traditional humoral theory and the more recent and controversial Paracelsian medicine." Selleck goes on to suggest that Donne subscribes to neither, given that "his contrast between the two models makes it quite clear that what he finds objectionable about the Galenic paradigm is its emphasis on digestion and concoction – that is, on the taking in of external 'correctives,' which then alter or become part of oneself," while "the 'chemic,' on the other hand, doesn't alter the self per se, but only removes what doesn't belong to it" (158). Hence Donne's poem subscribes to neither school but critiques both.

[23] Arthur W. Frank writes that "in 1623 John Donne's *Devotions* upon Emergent Occasions described his illness as a self-change of deepening religious faith." Frank may misread, though, in noting that Donne "was ahead of his time" in "presenting himself as a type of 'sick person' that did not yet exist" (39).

the Body" 216).[24] Accordingly, the author also recognizes that illness has advantages. Even as he also longs for "bodily restitution" in "Prayer XIX," Donne gives voice to the belief that affliction is a gift from a God who, though pleased "to glorifie thy selfe in a long exercise of my patience," does so "with an expectation of thy declaration of thy selfe in this my sicknesse" (46). Given the early modern reciprocity of physical and spiritual health – let alone Donne's status as ordained priest and Dean of St. Paul's – the *Devotions'* author ministers his body as well as soul. Donne may at times explicitly champion learned medicine's cause, but he cannot and does not grant the physician sole rule over his disease. Offering a patient's perspective on the emotion that is also the physicians' instrument of persuasion, Donne in "Meditation VI" observes "the physician with the same diligence as he the disease," through which, he says, "I see he fears." The physicians' sensibly discernible fear exacerbates his own, causing the patient to "fear with him." However much fear may belong to the patient who now insists that "I overtake him, I overrun him, in his fear, and I go the faster, because he makes his pace slow; I fear the more," the physician's trepidation exacerbates: "because he disguises his fear," maintains Donne, "I see it with the more sharpness, because he would not have me see it" (13).

The physician may also fear, but his profession demands that he command the emotion in a way the patient cannot. Unlike the sufferer, "he knows that his fear shall not disorder the practice and exercise of his art, but he knows that my fear may disorder the effect and working of his practice." Repeating the "fear" that is Donne's topic affirms its potential to bring about an undesirable "disorder" nevertheless. Confirming the interconnection of mind and body understood also by the medical practitioner, Donne writes of their proportional correspondence in Galenic terms: "As the ill affections of the spleen complicate and mingle themselves with every infirmity of the body," he observes, "so doth fear insinuate itself in every action or passion of the mind" (13). One must be careful to discern between actual illness, both physical and psychological, though it may not be easy to do so in a context and an author that equally evince what Selleck calls the "persistent presence" of Donne's deeply "humoral selfhood" (150). Accordingly, fear can bring about unhealthy imaginings as well as worsen the actual physical conditions. Just "as wind in the body will counterfeit

[24] Though Donne's *Devotions* may in some ways represent the tradition of protestant meditation, Mary Arshagouni Papazian complicates their generic status. "Although Donne may well make use of Protestant meditative techniques," Papazian argues, "this tradition fails not only to explain fully its overall structure but also to account for the emotional twists and turns experienced by the speaker during the course of his illness, arguably the essence of the work's affective power" (608).

any disease, and seem the stone, and seem the gout," writes Donne, so emotions can bring forth the appearance of illness, for "fear will counterfeit any disease of the mind" (13).

Hinting at patient agency through a mimicking fear beyond the capacity of the physicians' discourse to control, Donne also suggests its curative possibilities. Invoking in "Prayer VI" the Judeo-Christian belief that fear can benefit the soul, Donne writes,

> And therefore, though I pretend to no other degree of wisdom, I am abundantly rich in this, that I lie here possessed with that fear which is thy fear, both that this sickness is thy immediate correction, and not merely a natural accident, and therefore fearful, because it is a fearful thing to fall into thy hands; and that this fear preserves me from all inordinate fear, arising out of the infirmity of nature, because thy hand being upon me, thou wilt never let me fall out of thy hand. (15)

Donne's suffering bears testament to a God who is actually paying attention to him, and illness is no mere "natural accident" but, as Taylor and others would have it, an oxymoronic yet thankfully received mark of divine favour. As with the physician-authored texts, fear in Donne's may belong to the patient more than it does the physician; in the case of the *Devotions*, however, it is a fear that may be ultimately desirable, with advantages expressed in a paradoxical tautology of fear that "preserves me from all inordinate fear." Though aware of its physical dangers, the devotional Donne in the end has nothing to fear.

Replicating and resisting the physicians' emotional appeals, fear in Donne's *Devotions* further reveals what Selleck describes as his "conscious engagement with the paradigms and practices of humoral medicine." Making clear that "Galenic conceptions of health and disease" may "also suggest less rigid distinctions between self and world than modern medical theory" (150–51),[25] Donne also confirms that the physicians' hegemony was predicated on an epistemology that could not wholly support their

[25] Selleck makes a similar point in observing that "Donne's humoral imagery not only challenges the widespread view of his own 'individualism,' but also complicates recent critical discussions of Renaissance selfhood in general" (150). That Donne's medical rhetoric needs to be read within a larger cultural context Goldberg also makes clear in his seminal article on the *Devotions*. As much as we may value Donne's ingenuity, he is the product of a culture that, Goldberg reminds us, attached less value to "personal idiosyncracies" than "traditional themes" and views (507). In his exploration of "the commonplaces which lie at the center of Donne's understanding of the meaning of his illness" (507), Goldberg surveys numerous manuals and prayer books to show how Donne engages in the "traditional dilemma of the relationship of sickness to sin and salvation" (509), and is thus led from an examination of the self to one of the human condition and, concomitantly, to the desire for alacrity in physical adversity.

subjugating demands. His engagement with the discourse of "medicine in general and medical semiotics in particular" as well as the "discourse of affliction" in the *Devotions*, as Stephen Pender argues, in many ways attests to Donne's profound understanding of early modern medicine ("Essaying the Body" 217–19).[26] The example of a canonical author conversant with the language and knowledge of learned medicine despite a lack of formal training is, I would add, usefully illustrative of how even those who could not count themselves among the medical elite might also engage its discourse in complex, nuanced, and sometimes contradictory ways.

[26] Readers of the *Devotions* have identified the influences and ideas of Hippocrates, Aristotle, Galen, and Paracelsus in Donne's medical thought (Pender, "Essaying the Body" 218 n. 12). "Like an early modern physician," writes Pender, "Donne presses the body into epistemological service: to anatomise and read effects is to begin to discern causes, to know the sick body is to begin to know the sick soul" ("Essaying the Body" 230–31).

PART II

The Woman Writer

CHAPTER 4

"Publishing Those Truthes"
Women and Affliction

Because "such business is accompanied with much ease," advises Nicholas Fonteyn's *The Womans Doctor* (1652), and lest they worsen constitutions already "much weakned" by the "immoderate flowing" of the blood's "purest portion," women were "made to stay at home, and to looke after Houshold employments" (25). Constrained by the "monethly Courses" assigned by "provident Nature" (Fonteyn 1), women were further inconvenienced by wombs that bred not only the "convulsions, epilepsies, apoplexies, palseyes, hecticke fevers, dropsies, [and] malignant ulcers" John Sadler identifies in *The Sick Womans Private Looking-Glasse* (1636), but also "no disease so ill but may procede from the evill quality of it" ("The Epistle Dedicatory" n. pag.). Suggesting something of the challenge the afflicted woman faced in an age when the very act of speaking risked proving the "evill quality" Sadler insists upon, it has been argued that even the latter-day woman who writes about, through, or from illness must pay particular attention to fashioning "her own moral style, her own *ethos*" in the face of a culture that remains deeply misogynist (Baumlin and Baumlin 255).[1] Given that her casting to "patient type" was predicated on the feminine body's "evill quality," the potential to fashion a credible "moral style" in the face of illness would have been even more dramatically curtailed for the

[1] That women's voices were actively curtailed by some deep-seated notions about gender long supported by authority of all kinds has been amply demonstrated and, as we have seen in Chapter 3, early modern medical rhetoric worked to constrain women in practice as well as in theory. Early modern women were further inhibited by a general lack of education. As David Cressy has shown, not every reader in Tudor and Stuart England could also write, and "many people who are counted as illiterate because they could not write their names may in fact have had some ability to read" (142). The women who are the subject of this chapter were, however, writing at a time when women's literacy rates were on the upswing. Cressy also argues that great strides were made in the seventeenth century, proposing that a 90 per cent illiteracy rate among women in the century's early years that was reduced, at least in London, to 52 per cent by the 1690s (146). (See also Cressy's landmark book, *Literacy and the Social Order: Reading and Writing in Tudor and Stuart England* [Cambridge: Cambridge University Press, 1980]).

early modern woman.[2] In a Galenic context that, as Selleck puts it, "sees what we call 'personality' as a function of the body" (152), however, it may also be that the voices of women otherwise cast to sick, disordered type were not always silenced but sometimes enabled by illnesses that justified and effected a corresponding rebellion of mind.

Undertaking what might otherwise be avoided in fear of bold, presumptuous, and decidedly unfeminine behaviour, women who wrote about illness prove keenly aware of how affliction might work to persuasive effect. Paying particular attention to fashioning the good character on which their credibility relied, the work of authors from Royalist Lady Anne Halkett to shipwright's daughter and Fifth Monarchy Baptist Anna Trapnel points to a number of ways a culturally understood interdependence of mind, body, and spirit could work to rhetorical advantage. Writing from the patient's perspective, Halkett finds such advantage in illness-enabled confession, while the bed-bound Trapnel, chronically ill An Collins, and eponymous deliverer of *Elizas Babes* find in religion the means of positing their own bold critiques of the Cromwellian regime. Though essayist Mary Astell sees no such advantage in suffering, she does acknowledge that bodily affliction can serve mind and spirit through the reasoned preparation its inevitability demands; like Halkett and the Interregnum writers, Astell is able also to challenge gendered notions of behaviour because she foregrounds the scripture with which every believer was mandated to engage. Drawing on the discourse of religion, the rhetoric of women who wrote of afflictions bodily and spiritual thus aligns with that of the physician–clerics as well as clergymen such as Timothy Rogers and Richard Baxter, whose first-hand accounts of illness question the efficacy of learned medicine and affirm the importance of tending first and foremost to the soul. Sometimes amending as they participated in the dominant discourses of their day, early modern women can be seen also to engage a self-fashioning rhetoric akin to that of learned medicine as they work to forge a feminine self of "her own moral style" and "her own *ethos.*"

Lady Anne Halkett may have authored her memoir with no eye to dissemination, yet she did not write her story without an audience in mind.[3]

[2] The persuasive challenges ill women faced are not, however, so distinct from those encountered today. Modern medicine may command an understanding of female physiology much different from that of the early moderns but, Judy Segal finds in her study of illness as argument, physicians may yet focus on assigning "patient types." Likened to the nineteenth century's willfully incurable "hysterical malingerer," Segal proposes, patients who suffer from diseases such as fibromyalgia, a chronic and multi-symptomatic condition whose victims are most often female, may be particularly subject to typecasting by the illness that defines them.

[3] Halkett's memoir may have served as "the basis of a short biography published in Edinburgh in 1701" but, according to Ezell, it did not earlier circulate as a form of "scribal publication," there is "no

On the contrary, as Margaret Ezell argues, Halkett engaged a larger literary culture as she produced the autobiography Mary Ellen Lamb styles as both "tragicomedy and romance" (81). In early modern culture, participating in the literary meant also engaging the rhetorical, a necessity especially for one whose romantic misadventures might otherwise prove her undoing. Given that "central rhetorical motive for her writing," as Judith Kearns notes, turns out to be the "defense of her virtue" (341), Halkett's intently self-fashioning narrative is in large measure shaped by what Sandra Findley and Elaine Hobby read as "the twin motives of confession and vindication" (17). Given that women of Halkett's day were famously urged to chastity, silence, and obedience, both the writing of the autobiography and the behaviour it describes, as Kearns observes, go a long way to disrupt "any naïve notions that women of her time were entirely constrained by dominant cultural stereotypes" (341). Recounting a tale that might prove her disobedient and unchaste, Halkett's defence of her own virtue is well served by the account of her affliction and recovery. Illness may prove corruption, but it also serves to fashion her virtue and her authority and, in so doing, confirms the parallel understanding that language artfully used can go a long way toward negotiating – and also relieving – afflictions of mind, body, and spirit.

Halkett's memoir is particularly intent on defending what was nearly undone by her relationship with a married man who, she maintains, "had abused me in pretending his wife was dead" (32).[4] Struck by a truth made evident, Halkett fell ill by a cause equally inflicting mind, body, and spirit. If the suffering that came upon learning that she had been dallying with a liar, scoundrel, and eventual turncoat were not enough, Halkett's health was further compromised by other bad news. Had the event "comme singly itt had beene enough to have tried the strengh [sic] of all the religion and virtue I had," she professes, but was too much to bear at a time "surrounded with misfortunes." So affected that she was near death, Halkett claims to have "fell so extreamely sicke that none expected life for mee" (32). Admitting that the misguided trust of love brought about her affliction while desiring to absolve herself of blame by claiming not to know

indication that Halkett showed her texts to others until shortly before her death," and her work did not appear in print until 1875. The circumstances of Halkett's autobiography thus "may not signal a maidenly avoidance of technology but a literary life engaged with print culture in interesting and complicated ways" ("Posthumous Publication" 215–17).

4 Halkett identifies her lover only as C.B., but he is understood to have been one Colonel Joseph Bampfield, "who seems," notes Kearns, to have been "by all accounts, save her own, a scoundrel," and one who would "eventually desert the Royalist cause" and proved "equally opportunistic in his personal life," thus leading Halkett to believe him a widower (340).

that her lover's wife yet lived, she extracted promises of letters later to be written on her behalf as she "lay waiting till my change should come" while "all was weeping about mee" (32–33). Certain of posthumously proving the full truth of the matter and thus assured of her reputation's safety, she waited for the death imminently "expected as the greatest good" as she for "some hours speechlese" lay (33). What she thought about while awaiting death's arrival Halkett does not yet reveal but promises soon to present an account of how she "employed that time" (33). Halkett thus uses her illness to emphasize her innocence in the affair and, by deferring the full account, holds focus on her suffering and her virtue while piquing the desire to learn what may have effected misfortune's reversal.[5]

We already know, of course, that Halkett was not permanently silenced. After those speechless hours, she finally "began to gape many times" and "found sencibly like a returne of my spiritts" (33). Mimed and shadowy it may be, but the return of some semblance of speech is in Halkett's account coincident or correlative with the return of her senses and spirits, and may even be causally linked. Urging the ill woman to rally, her female companion, Halkett writes, "came to mee and told mee if I saw another in that condition I could prescribe what was fit for them; and therefore itt were a neglect of duty if I did not use what meanes I thought might conduce to my recovery" (33). Persuaded by her companion's argument, Halkett complies and orders what she would have prescribed for another in the same state. Accordingly, she writes, "I called to Crew (who served mee) for itt, and with y[e] use of some cordials, I sencibly grew better" (33). Halkett's self-prescription, it turns out, outdoes the earlier recommendations of a local physician who, "being sicke" himself, could not attend her but "sent things" that "proved ineffectuall" (32) while her own remedy worked "to the satisfaction of all that was about mee" (33). Yet intent on emphasizing a virtue that encompasses patient acceptance, however, Halkett does not linger on her success. Confessing instead that "death at that time had beene extreamely welcome," she will neither lament rescue from its door, for "having intirely resigned myself up to the disposal of my gracious God," she maintains, "I could repine att nothing hee thought fit to do with mee, for I knew hee could make either life or death for my advantage" (33).

[5] "Appropriating the familiar conventions of the romance to her own rhetorical purposes" (Kearns 341) and intent on defending and demonstrating her own virtue, Halkett further displays a high degree of literary awareness evident also in her interest in creating narrative suspense and demonstrable understanding of literary genres. Lamb also argues that Halkett's *Memoirs* are both secular and sacred, though the work has been often read as akin to the religious meditations she also wrote (82) – a tendency that may say more about gendered expectations than the autobiography.

Halkett herself cannot profess to know which would have served her better; having fully expected and welcomed one outcome, she submits and is wholly prepared to recognize the advantages of the other. Quickly shifting to assert ready submission to divine will, Halkett abandons her own healing success in a *paraleptic* gesture that makes her point while serving a modest and therefore suitably feminine ethos.

Only after having worked to fashion an ethos both authoritative and virtuous does Halkett amend the explanation for her illness to confess that she had, in fact, committed a lie of omission. Though she claims to have believed her suitor's wife dead, she purports to have suppressed that knowledge in an earlier interaction, when she answered her sister's query about the affair with the indignant "Sure, you would nott have mee marry another woman's husband!" (34). It is not at first glance easy to comprehend why Halkett acknowledged her lover constrained by a wife instead of choosing simply to "say shee was dead," and hers is an odd response to the accusation of dallying with one she only later professes to have thought a widower. Halkett's maneuverings may, however, be more strategic than strange. Specious her explanation might be, but in suppressing knowledge that would have made her participation in the affair more acceptable to her sister, Halkett absolves herself of blame in the reader's eyes as she creates the opportunity to demonstrate humility as she goes on to confess a different offence.

Admitting to having been deservedly "inflicted for my disimulation" in not revealing that she had in fact believed her lover a widower, she claims to have "a thousand times" begged the pardon of a God who "requireth truth in the inward parts" (34). Halkett willingly admits not to the sin of outright fabrication but to the lesser lie of concealing her belief that the wife was in fact dead. Strategically, she does so while deflecting the implication of knowing adultery she earlier (and inexplicably) neglected to counter with her best evidence. Based as it is on the dubious claim that she chose not to reveal what she later professes to have believed, Halkett's account may not be very convincing, but it is significant that she does attempt to explain her lie-induced affliction by reasoned argument. Drawing attention away from implications of knowing adultery and toward deceit by omission, Halkett deploys the persuasion of logos to turn two sins to ethical advantage. Though she proves herself "neither silent nor obedient" (341), as Kearns puts it, Halkett's maneuvering leaves the "unchaste" of much greater offence an open question. Admitting deserved punishment for lying to herself as well as others, she displays the requisite modesty and humility in confessing a fault that (rhetorically at least) absolves her of knowing participation in an adulterous affair that may yet damage her future.

Following illness, recovery, and cause, her account takes up the Royalist lover. Equally attentive to logos and ethos, once she "began to recover," Halkett writes, her thoughts returned to the plight of the by-then-imprisoned man she worried might be condemned to death. Despite her "trouble and feares," she was "much suported one day by reading what fell outt to bee part of my morning devotion." The reading, she explains, was from "(Psa. 102, vers. 19,20: 'For hee hath lokked downe from ye height of his sanctuary; from heaven did the Lord behold the earth. To heare the groaning of the prisoner; to loose those that are apointed to death.')" Halkett commits no sinful lapse here, but "cannott omitt to mention this because itt was so seasonable a promise" and "was so asisted by faith to rely upon itt that in a manner itt overcame all my feares" (34). Halkett understands that it is not the words themselves but the recollections and emotions the Psalm evokes that bring about the peace that passeth understanding; she is able to find solace because of the poem's immediate relevance to her, an experience of illness and near-death that grants its pathos-invoking words "so seasonable a promise."

Writing of healing that encompasses body, mind, and spirit, Halkett demonstrates a nuanced understanding of the persuasion of rhetoric manifest in her attentiveness to its *entechnic* proofs. Recognizing the Psalm's pathos, Halkett aims also to move an audience she works to fashion through her recounted physical and psychological suffering. Declaring that "itt is nott to bee imagined by any pious, vertuous person" that she should have "such an odium cast" upon her for thinking "to marry a man that had a wife," she implies a reader whose virtue would not allow the condemnation of one who "abhorred the thought of such a crime." For this, she declares, "I am sure none could detest mee," especially those, she maintains within parentheses more amplifying than subordinating, "whose charity leads them to judge of others by themselves." The emphatically empathic aim of Halkett's aside is further reinforced with the also-parenthetical insistence on "how innocent so ever I was" that soon follows (35). Appealing to a presumed desire not to be thought lacking in piety or virtue, the unspoken premise of Halkett's pathos leads *enthymematically* to the conclusion that no judicious reader could therefore condemn her. Confessing one fault while deflecting blame for another, the reasoning of Halkett's logos works in the service of an ethos whose willing submission to divine will suggests a piety akin to that of her pathos-moved reader, her humility further evident in her willingness to tell but not trumpet a healing knowledge that surpasses the physician's. Finding advantage in suffering, Halkett's account of its causes and cures suggests something of at least one woman's knowing participation in an early modern rhetoric whose persuasive force shares much with that of the learned physicians.

Through the exigence of illness, the named but unidentified An Collins, the pseudonymous "Eliza," and the prophet Anna Trapnel also found opportunity to exercise their voices. Rather than inscribing themselves as types, however, all three ignore misogynist inscriptions of female physiology to find a measure of authorial as well as spiritual empowerment in writing from, about, or through bodily affliction. That they are able to do so has much to do with the religious orientation that, as Kenneth Burke has taught us, is deeply and inevitably rhetorical.[6] In a healing context where discourses medical and religious are predicated on an interconnected mind, body, and soul, their work in some ways also implies a vaguely felt sense of what researchers have recently begun to rediscover, that rhetoric is also an "uttering of healing words" (Baumlin and Baumlin 247). Persuading themselves as well as a potential or actual audience, Collins, Eliza, and Trapnel each deploy a rhetoric that, like Halkett's, appeals to the pathos of religious belief upheld by a logos predicated on the authority of scripture, both of which work to fashion the ethos on which their credibility depends.

Corroborating Fonteyn's stay-at-home advice, Collins's 1653 *Divine Songs and Meditacions* tells of an author "restrained from bodily employments" and bound "to a retired Course of life" because of lifelong affliction. Collins does not, however, reveal whether her retiredness responds to a like problem with "monethly Courses." Though hinting elsewhere about the nature of her malady, Collins remains undiagnosed, and a lack of textual evidence, together with the wealth of chronic illnesses thought to afflict early modern women, makes it difficult even to venture a guess.[7] More important than the identity of Collins's sickness, at any rate, is what she was able to discover because of it. Rather than debilitating her psyche along with her body, Collins tells us that her "seeming desolate condicion, proved to me most delightfull" in effecting a corresponding "inlargednesse of mind, and activity of spirit." A necessary confinement, it appears, enabled an "activity of spirit" that compelled her to become "affected to Poetry, insomuch that I proceeded to practise the same." The reciprocity

6 "The subject of religion," Burke writes, "falls under the head of rhetoric in the sense that rhetoric is the art of persuasion, and religious cosmogonies are designed, in the last analysis, as exceptionally thoroughgoing modes of persuasion" (*The Rhetoric of Religion* v).

7 Collins's specific illness is undetermined, but she does allude to some of its symptoms. Sarah E. Skwire observes that barrenness may be implied by the non-appearing "flowers" associated with menstruation and the lack of "hopefull bud" or "fruitfull bough" Collins refers to in "Another Song (The Winter of My Infancy)," while Sidney Gottlieb points to images that may hint at smallpox or an anatomical anomaly (219).

of writing and understanding soon became known to Collins, and the production of poetry thus "appeared unto me so amiable," she explains, spurring invention as it "enflamed my faculties, to put forth themselves, in a practise so pleasing" (1). The private comfort and intellectual inspiration Collins discovered through her illness-enabled writing gave rise to a voice that would soon become public and, despite her professions to the contrary, overtly and thoroughly rhetorical.[8]

Neither Trapnel nor Eliza, however, appears to have been chronically ill. In her 1652 collection of poetry and meditations, *Eliza's Babes: Or the Virgin's Offerings* invokes a familiar trope as she describes her "Souls sweet Babes" that "do bring no pain" ("On Marriage" 42, line 11). Eliza likens literary production with childbirth that, notes Elizabeth Clarke, is like "ejaculation" in its association "with discourses which stress the agency of God and the passivity of the human author in composition" (222).[9] Eliza may claim her poetic offspring as her own, but figures an ethos that may be proud in ownership but humble in deferring to divine inspiration. Given that she repeatedly indicates that she had no actual children, Eliza's simultaneously self-effacing and self-determining trope does not encompass any literal experience of childbirth. She does, however, take up affliction in the consecutive poems "Being in Paine" (48) and "Being taken with a sudden pain on the Day appointed for God's publick Service" (48–49). "Let not this pain," she writes in the latter, "Lord, deter me"

From publick offering praise to thee.
Though private prayers may pleasing bee
From others, and as well from me.
But publick blessings thou giv'st me,
And publick praise I'de offer thee.
(lines 1–6)

[8] Collins claims that her volume was intended for "private use" and not "publick view" ("The Discourse" lines 15–17), yet other evidence suggests that she did not write without the public in mind. A gesture not exclusive to women, "private use" Henry Scudder also claims for the origins of his 1631 *Christian's Daily Walk*, a work that is "now (through importunity) published for the common good." (For a fuller discussion of the public and private in Collins, Eliza, and Trapnel, see Bennett, "Negotiating the Public and the Private: Rhetoric and Women's Poetry in Interregnum England" (*Rhetor* 4 [2011]).

[9] The metaphor hearkens from antiquity, and is familiar in the work of poets like Philip Sidney and Samuel Daniel. The offspring metaphor is, however, not exclusive to verse any more than it belongs only to women. In *The Cause and Cure of a Wounded Conscience* (1649), Fuller even genders his production, specifying that "this Booke is my eldest Off-spring, which had it beene a Sonne, (I mean, had it been a Worke of Masculine beauty and bignesse) it should have waited as a Page in Dedication to his *Honour* … But finding it to be of the weaker sexe, little in strength and low in stature, may it be admitted (*Madam*) to attend on your *Ladiship*, his *Honours* sister" ("Epistle Dedicatory to Frances Mannours," dated January 25, 1646, Sig. $A3_v$).

Unlike Collins, Eliza makes clear that she means not to praise only in private.[10] That "publick praise" is more suited than "private prayers" to giving thanks for "publick blessings" she further confirms in "To the Reader," where she maintains that her reluctance to send her *Babes* "into the world" was thoroughly overcome by her desire to give "publique thankes, for such infinite and publque [sic] favours" ("To the Reader" 57–58). That she was prevented from doing so because of a "pain" suggests that Eliza's physical malady was not only the poem's impetus but also the means of strengthening her rhetorical resolve, the forced restraint of unexpected illness making her more determined to make "publick offering."

In the self-authored testimony preceding the dictated prophecies of Trapnel's 1654 *The Cry of a Stone*, the author writes also of an affliction that gave rise to her public voice. It all began "seven years ago," she explains, when "being visited with a feaver, given over by all for dead, the Lord then gave me faith to believe from that Scripture" (Sig. $A2_r$/3). If "women's authority as spiritual leaders" in the seventeenth century was, as Phyllis Mack claims, grounded in "their achievement of complete self-transcendence" (5), it may be that the persuasiveness evident in Trapnel's subsequent popularity was largely achieved not through a physical but a psychic anomaly, the famous trances that granted her spiritual authority. Regardless, Trapnel's testimony makes clear that it was the actual "feaver" that fortified her faith and established her credibility in a culture in which "bodily weakness," Diane Purkiss notes, also "acted as a signifier for prophetic empowerment" (145). Like Collins and Eliza, Trapnel presents affliction as authorial catalyst, and it is from that illness that she fashions an ethos that allowed her to speak publicly and, in her case at least, even be taken seriously.[11] In one way or another, privately suffered illness is the vehicle through which all three women find and articulate a rhetoric whose devotional orientation works to justify the speech of women who would, they equally imply, otherwise choose silence.

[10] The pseudonym may indicate that "Eliza" meant to remain out of the public eye, and she confirms as much in "To a friend at Court," where she claims to relish "sweet retirednesse" that "quiet thought contenteth" (lines 4–5), and in "My pleasing Life," where she praises the "sweet quiet, sweet obscurity" that "best pleaseth" (lines 1–2). In other poems, however, Eliza belies her professed wish for "retirednesse" in boldly writing "To the King" and "To Generall Cromwell."

[11] Trapnel's authority is, of course, mediated by her scribe. Trapnel's self-styled "'Relator' wrote down only as much of her oral and extempore compositions as he could, given his 'very slow and unready hand' (Sig. $A2_v$) and a frequent 'press of people in the Chamber' (19), so we cannot know with certainty how closely the text corresponds with Trapnel's speech," and "her amanuensis also regularly intervenes, contextualizing and interpreting her words as well as voicing his own opinions" (Bennett, "Negotiating the Public and the Private" 4). The resulting ethos is nevertheless predicated on Trapnel's illness, and *The Cry of a Stone* is presented as the product of a female voice.

Collins, Eliza, and Trapnel also imply benefits to their physical as well as spiritual well-being, recognizing with the ancients that the right use of language could have the "salutary effect on physical health" (5) more recently confirmed by James Pennebaker's studies of language and therapeutic writing.[12] They surely also shared the sense of disruption and disorder brought about by two recent civil wars and an Interregnum context that in many ways saw their world indeed turned upside down, the king displaced by an army general, and a once-relatively united church splintered into a dizzying array of factions and sects. The dominant narrative within which Collins, Eliza, and Trapnel locate their experiences of illness was, as a result, in many ways nationalistic, but was above all one of intense and ubiquitous religious devotion. That devotion extended to personal obligation expressed by Trapnel in her imperative urging to "let thy servants now be of a publique spirit" (Sig. $F3_v$/38). Albeit in different ways, the work of all three strived to make discursive sense out of Interregnum chaos.

The resulting attempt to negotiate a public discourse informed by religion and shaped by rhetoric Eliza makes clear in preemptive response to anticipated detractors. "Let them know," she declares, "that if they did rightly apprehend the infinite mercies of God to them, they could not be silent." Justifying her God-given right to speak, Eliza does "them" one better as she goes on, "And if they doe not thinke the mercies of God worth publique thankes; I doe, and therefore I will not be ashamed" ("To the Reader" Sig. $A3_r$). Devotional tribute is a Christian obligation and not a mere prerogative, and Eliza insists that shamefulness does not accrue to those willing to give public thanks, including women, but to those whose failure to do so suggests they believe God undeserving. Moreover, the example Gideon Burton invokes to define *aetiologia* as the "figure of reasoning by which one attributes a cause for a statement or claim made, often as a simple relative clause of explanation" (*Silva Rhetoricæ*) sounds remarkably akin to Eliza's: "So, as much as in me is," reads the passage from Romans, "I am ready to preach the gospel to you that are at Rome also. For I am not ashamed of the gospel of Christ: for it is the power of God unto salvation to every one that believeth; to the Jew first, and also to the Greek" (1:15–16). Alluding to a text as familiar as it is rhetorically aware, Eliza reiterates gospel truth as personal belief.

[12] Pennebaker and his colleagues have extensively researched the relationship of writing and healing; their work is also complemented by "several dozen studies from multiple laboratories around the world" demonstrating the positive health effects of writing on subjects in varying occupations, social classes, and ethnic groups (Pennebaker 5).

More explicit about paying verbal tribute, Trapnel claims divinely ordained duty with the prefatory assertion that "the Lord made use of me for the refreshing of afflicted and tempted ones." Though Trapnel here refers to the affliction of soul, her claim to effects both "inwardly and outwardly" (*Cry* Sig. $A2_r$/3) also implies that her words brought some aid to the body. Much as the history of "self-help," as Porter puts it, recognizes that "initiatives" and "power" have "often come from" and "frequently rested with" sufferers ("The Patient's View" 175), so Trapnel's comes not from the discourses of religion and medicine but the spoken words that were, for reasons of incapacity or dramatic necessity, recorded by another. Trapnel does, however, claim to write "from her own hand" in the later 1654 *Report and Plea*. Recounting her preaching journey to Cornwall and subsequent trial and imprisonment in Bridewell, she may agree to being "unworthy to be compared with any of the holy men or women reported of in the Scripture," but insists that she is nevertheless fit to speak because "Christ lives in me." Like Eliza, Trapnel claims God-given authority in shaping a moral and spiritual ethos sometimes upheld as superior to that of an audience that either neglects or is not moved by devotional obligation to speak. Doing what she says she will not do in the process of saying so, however, she indulges in the *paraleptic* as she goes on to claim an intention not to speak out against the malice of others against her. "The Lord knows," Trapnel insists, that "I would not reach out tongue, hand nor pen, to right my self, or to seek restauration of my loss." Trapnel thus manages to rebuke her detractors while claiming to rise above them: "I wave that," she concludes, "such a thing is below my spirit" (*Report* Sig. $A2_v$). In denying an aim to right or restore what she has suffered or lost, Trapnel professes to speak not in self-service, and her indignant dismissal of such an intent serves an ethos whose faults are excused by proclaimed service to the Christian good.

Collins's self-effacing rhetoric makes itself known from from the beginning, in "The Preface" that readily admits that "sounder judgments" may "declare / The ground of Truth more in a Gospel-way" (lines 85–86) and "more plainly shew the path-way to Salvacion" (line 91). Yet she too professes a religious duty that excuses what would otherwise entail a marked breach of social decorum. Modesty, she admits, "cannot prevail to hinder me, / From publishing those Truthes I do intend" (lines 92–93). Holding devotional duty over gendered notions of decorum, Collins does so by invoking the faithful obligation of religion. That she participates fully in its discourse is evident in that she, like Eliza, not only writes squarely within the tradition of the religious lyric but also, as Ann Hurley explains, "cites scripture directly" and follows "prose traditions in listing the relevant scriptural verse in the margins of her verse" (234). Collins may expressly reject the "colours" that "glose" as akin to "cloth most foully staind" ("A Song composed in time of the Civill Warr" 61, lines 21 and 24) and expose theological sophists who aim "by Elocution / And Hellish Logick to traduce" ("Another Song" 64, lines 22–23), but she also takes up the persuasive conventions of the tradition in which she is thoroughly immersed. Like all religious writers, she aims to relate "the ground of Truth" ("The Discourse" 30, line 708) she has come to understand, and hopes that her appeal to the Christian soul shall "full perswasion see" and thereby share her "strength of Faith" ("The Discourse" 26, lines 566–67).

Giving voice to the evangelical belief in professing what one has discovered, Eliza, Trapnel, and Collins's self-fashioning depends on reiterating the terms of a larger narrative. In doing so, all three necessarily express "the commitments inherited from previous 'speech acts' publicly performed" that, as Thomas B. Farrell argues, characterize the rhetorical (119). Making visible those inherited commitments in a public performance, Collins aims "former workes to vindicate" more "than any new concepcion to relate" ("The Preface" lines 13–14). In vindicating "former workes," Collins defers to a textual tradition she promises only to verify; at the same time, however, she does so by laying claim to the knowledge necessary to do so.[13] Uttering through illness-enabled writing an intuitive "got by heart" belief in "sacred principles" ("The Discourse" 14, line 208) within the terms of an established discourse, her words thus further imply rhetoric's value in treating the self. Writing to heal oneself is a mere step away from using language to heal others and, "if thou wilt be importunate in prayer," as William Fenner urges in *Practicall Divinitie* (1647), one should also "labour to reform thy houshold" (107). That they believed they could reform through writing both Eliza and Collins make clear, while it may also be that Trapnel, as Hilary Hinds proposes, not only understood the particular "power of written language" to heal the spirit but may also have recognized "the physical effect it can have on the reader" (126). The compulsion of religious duty may justify the voices of Collins, Eliza, and Trapnel, but the means for doing so may come only because they also write about and through the healing power of devotion in their private lives and, in Trapnel's case at least, anticipate physical as well as spiritual repair.

[13] Critics most often read the *humilitas topos* deployed by women writers from Mary Sidney Herbert to Anne Bradstreet as sincere expressions of modesty and marginality. Patricia Pender, however, resists the "familiar story of women's gendered oppression," reading "modesty rhetoric" instead "as the very mark of literariness as it circulates among early modern protocols of textual modesty and authority" (3). Hence such gestures also confirm women's full participation in rhetorical culture.

Understanding that her affliction is "by divine Providence" ("To the Reader" 1), Collins accepts suffering without complaint. Fortitude may even have transformed physical sickness to "delightfull" condition and, because "it pleased God to give me Writing," she is not ungrateful for the providential kindness arising from a wounding dispensation. As Taylor puts it, illness is "a little image of the state of blessed Souls" (109), and Collins understood as well as Donne that her soul may have been the greatest beneficiary of her illness-enabled writing. Though not without bodily benefit, "the helps I had therein were small," Collins admits, but she may have gained more than physical relief could bring: "the least grain of the increase of *grace*," as Younge writes in offering *A sovereign antidote against all grief*, "is more worth, then can be equalled with whole pounds of *bodily vexation*." In the end, Collins may not want to alleviate physical suffering altogether if she believes, with Younge, that those "whole pounds of *bodily vexation*" should be taken as "tokens and pledges of *Gods love* and favour, who loves his Children so, as not to make *wantons* of them" (166). Collins's illness may, in fact, be her means of salvation, for sometimes "sicknesse is a messenger sent from a chastising Father," writes Taylor, and "none but suffering, humble, and patient persons can go to heaven" (121–24).[14]

However purposeful, illness is not always a welcome corrective. "Lord, if my sin produce my paine," Eliza pleads, "pray let me never sin againe" ("Being in Paine" 48, lines 1–2). The undesirable consequence of misbehaviour, "pain is grievous unto me," she goes on,

> And sin is hatefull unto thee.
> Let me not do what troubleth thee,
> And thou'lt not send what grieve shall me.
> (lines 3–6)

[14] The "blessed state" of the paradise that belonged to Adam cannot, of course, compare with the paradise to come. In the song titled "Having Prayed for, and made much mention of the Merchants, she Sings the following Hymn to them," Trapnel extols what is to come over what has passed:

> Of that old Paradise, before
> A Christ a new one brings,
> Which shall abide for evermore,
> Where thine shall in it sing.
> Oh how greatly then are those Saints
> Established by thee,
> That hast a rest brought forth to them,
> Where they shall alwaies be.
> Oh it is much more better, sure
> Then Adams state before;
> Oh here is one that is so strong,
> None can it rend nor tore. (Sig. D4v/32)

Eliza makes clear her desire to avoid affliction, but she is ambiguous about whether avoiding "what troubleth thee" or "what grieve shall me" is more important. Physical pain for its own sake is not something she will suffer gladly, "But if my patience Lord thou tryest," she also affirms,

> If I will bear, what thou applyest,
> To cure the malady of sin,
> Cease not my pain, but send't again;
> For pain I rather would endure,
> Then grieve thine eyes of light so pure.
> (lines 7–12)

Eliza is willing to suffer physicially if it enables spiritual clarity, and pain is welcome if it means to cure as well as punish "the malady of sin." Like the "one in ten" who has returned "a cleansed Leaper," the poet recognizes "the infinite mercies of God" and takes it on gospel authority that she must not "be silent" ("To the Reader" Sig. A3_r).[15]

Enabling the "faith to believe from that Scripture" (*Cry* Sig. A2_r), Trapnel also attributes her fever to godly purpose. Yet merely "submitting to God's will in suffering," as Henry Hammond writes in his 1659 discussion of the Psalms, may suggest "but a very moderate degree of Christian fortitude" (493). Trapnel, however, exceeds the merely moderate when, according to her self-appointed scribe, she was later "seized upon by the Lord" and fell into her famous twelve-day trance. "The first five days neither eating nor drinking any thing more or less" but "a very little toast in small Bear" (*Cry* Sig. A_r/1), Trapnel did not merely submit but perhaps chose also to "prove fasting to be a Christian duty" as Henry Scudder's *The Christians Daily Walke in Holy Securitie and Peace* (1631) argues in a brief passage supported by no fewer than five scriptural references:

> Our Lord and Saviour said, [Mat. 9. 15] that his Disciples after his departure from them should fast; & giveth direction unto all touching [Mat. 6. 16 17] priuate fasts. The Apostle [1 Cor. 7. 5] speaketh of the husbands and wiues abstaining from the marriage bed, that they might giue themselvs to fasting and prayer: And wee haue the practise of the [Act· 13. 2, 3 Act. 14. 23] Apostles againe and again for publike fasts. (72)

According to Scudder, fasting brings advantages to both "husbands and wiues," but it may be that, as Hinds proposes, women especially needed

[15] See Luke 17.12–18

to provide the "empty vessels" that granted "the signifying capabilities of words and bodies" (144).[16]

It was also universally understood that "for patience, for Christian fortitude, for resignation, or conformity to the Divine will, it is necessary in the state of vertues that some portion and period of our lives be assigned to passive graces," but, Taylor also confirms, God has "given us the whole stage of our life to exercise all the active vertues" (124). According to Taylor, active virtue demands priority through "the whole stage of our life," and entails more than Hammond's merely "submitting to God's will in suffering." Made visible as the fasting that was as crucially persuasive as the words she spoke, the success of Trapnel's ethos depended as much on the signs provided by her body as the language of her mind. It may be that "because rhetorical proficiency *was not* expected from a woman that Trapnel's words were considered credible," as Maria Magro claims (421), but those who "slight thy handmaid," *The Cry of a Stone* avers, are also mistaken to "say these are Convulsion-fits, and Sickness, and diseases that make thy handmaid to be in weakness."[17] On the contrary, those who do so fail to recognize that persuasion comes also through the body, and "know not the pouring forth of thy Spirit, for that makes the body to crumble, and weakens nature." If they could read aright, they would understand that "in these extraordinary workings" the Lord "intendest to shew what is coming forth" (Sig. $D3_r$/29).

Trapnel's body also provided the means of showing what amounts to her own shadowy Resurrection: "After two days I will revive thee," the Saviour told her, and "the third day I will raise thee up, and thou shalt live in my sight." As divinely sanctioned exegete, however, Trapnel allows

16 Narveson notes that "treatises on fasting similarly draw the lines of influence from body to soul. Purification of the body conditions the spirits that knit body and soul together" (323). Yet the very public setting of Trapnel's trance may have aimed to ensure that her body reached full signifying potential. Jane Shaw suggests that Trapnel saw her fast-induced suffering as a physical testament to piety (109), while William Tyndall, in his biography of John Bunyan, writes of Trapnel that "the sickness which fell upon her as upon Bunyan *was* more sociable than his; for she admitted the public to the infirmary of her body and soul, and displayed her curious motions, delirium and fits of ravishment and palsy to the fascinated and devout" (qtd. in Berg and Berry 48).

17 Phyllis Mack argues that Trapnel lived in "a culture in which spiritual suffering and communication with the divine were viewed as real, indeed normative experiences," and that visionary women were thus "far from being a marginalized, hysterical fringe group in seventeenth-century society" (93). Trapnel may, however, have worked harder than Mack's view indicates. Magro implies as much in suggesting the need to call upon all at her disposal, relying on "language and body work together to convince the spectator that Trapnel is the 'real thing' " (415). That a carefully fashioned ethos, as Segal notes, is just as important to the sick person today, given that "a claim that is substantially weak (logos)," she says, "may be rehabilitated when the speaker shows him/herself to be trustworthy (ethos)" (237), suggests how important it would have been to early modern women in illness.

her own spin on Christ's promise, "which two days were two weeks," she explains in temporal equivalence, "that I should lye in that feaver, and that very time that it took me, that very hour it should leave me, and I should rise and walk, which was accordingly" (*Cry* Sig. $A2_r/3$). Manifest most perfectly where the "Word was made flesh" (John 1.14), the uttering of healing words finds evidence in the gospel, where "Jesus went about all the cities and villages, teaching in their synagogues, and preaching the gospel of the kingdom, and healing every sickness and every disease among the people" (Matt. 9.35). Teaching and preaching, both of which depend on rhetorical skill for their success, are linked in Matthew's formulation as two parts in a trinity of divine action, the third component of which is healing. Where Christ is concerned, the healing utterance is not explicitly coextant with the endless cycle of injury and repair set in motion by the Word, but mirrors the eloquence that is the Father's.

For His lesser images, however, eloquence heals to the extent that, Prideaux avers, it "is a Logicall kind of Rhetorick, to be used in Prayer, Preaching or Conference; to the glory of God, and the convincing, instructing, and strengthening our brethren" (Sig. $A2_r$). In all three aims, the rhetoric of Collins, Eliza, and Trapnel meets the standards of Prideaux's "sacred eloquence." Or, as Collins puts it in "A Song demonstrating The vanities of Earthly things" (41–42), the learning of geometry, geography, and astronomy may lead one to "mis of heaven and heavenly blis" (line 31), while "they that delight in Divinity" and are "exquisite in Theology, / Much heavenly comfort in this life may gain" (lines 33–35). Engaging the religious in a passage that follows her prose rendering of "Psalme 56. Vers. 10," Eliza makes clear the kind of words she writes: "And when you read these lines," she advises in *antimetabolic* form, "mistake not a Divine affection, for a Poetical fancy; for I affect not to express my fancy, but I would have my fancy express my affection" (Sig. $A4_r/1$). Bringing the latter "affection" back to the root "affect," the formal tautology of *affect / fancy / fancy / affection* underscores the interdependence of the imaginative "fancy" that brings a "Divine affection" too easily mistaken for yet simultaneously brought into being by the poet's "affect." The tension between the nominal "affection" and verbal "affect" is, of course, addressed with the "not" that does not negate but underscores the too-ready mistaking of one for another. Achieving in form as well as content the "necessary harmony between language and truth" Hinds finds in Trapnel (125), Collins, Eliza, and Trapnel demonstrate the understanding shared with the Levellers to come, the recognition that no matter how despised or dismissed, "in the real world," as Rachel Foxley proposes, "rhetoric might be truth's only effective ally" (282).[18] Writing with "convincing, instructing, and strengthening" aim "to the glory of God," they prove full (if reluctant) participants in the "Logicall kind of Rhetorick" that defines sacred eloquence.

Claiming to speak only "to advance Christ, and not for any by-end" (*Report* 6), Trapnel may profess to reject a political discourse that exploits the religious, but she is not averse to doing the same. Participating in a larger discourse does not, however, also mean that they must faithfully replicate its terms. Though drawing from the Old Testament as well as the gospels and especially from Revelation, Trapnel's work is most striking not for slavish imitation but an imaginative re-visioning that amplifies and explicates the source that is scripture's most cryptic book. Inspiring the assurance Hobbes describes in his *Art of Rhetoric* as "arising from an imagination that the help is near, or the evil afar off" ("Of Assurance" 56), Trapnel's pathos appeals to the inner life of her audience as she figures forth the workings of her imagination. Fashioned by the "good words, great allegories, and high expressions" her prophecies offer in lieu of the more usual "vaine conceits, vaine speculations, and high notions," Trapnel holds up for imitation a "publique spirit" that might empower the godly also to "flie high above the Skies" (*Cry* Sig. $F3_v$/38). In this and other ways, the persuasive force of *enargeia* offers the means of providing relief to the "afflicted and tempted" (*Cry* Sig. $A2_r$/3). Vividly displaying the rhetorical virtue Aristotle calls bringing-before-the-eyes, Trapnel figures an endless parade of images familiar and fresh. As with the horns of Revelation that become "four Powers," they most often come with a presently relevant interpretation. Three of those horns are obviously faulty, the named "Bishops," the army "endeavouring to get up a Mount" that "had joyned to it an head," the Parliament "consisting of many Men" whose "fair pretences of love to all under all forms" lie "broken and scattered," while the fourth seems fair. The last may be "short" but is "full of variety of Colours" and tempting with its "sparkling red and white" and "great swelling words and great offers of kindness." This fair-seeming

[18] Foxley notes that "'rhetoricall' appears as a pejorative term in Leveller writing alongside 'scholastical', 'sophisticall', 'syllogisticall', 'glosses', 'long set speeches', and so on. Almost anything that smacks of scholarliness can thus be bracketed with rhetoric. The Levellers critique genuine elements of rhetorical theory, but they also denounce 'rhetoric' in the general sense in which we often understand the word today" (270–71). That may be so, but they do indulge in a great deal of rhetoric of their own.

fourth, it turns out, is the church that, by colluding with government and opposing the Fifth Monarchy Baptists, offers only the semblance of worth (*Cry* Sig. $A3_r$/5).[19]

Trapnel's visions may be cryptic but her arguments are far from subtle. Near the end of *The Cry of a Stone*, Trapnel offers not an allegorical critique of the episcopacy, army, government, or church, but a notably allusive defence of the lay prophesier. Beginning with objections *erotemically* ventriloquized, "You will say," the speaker anticipates, "have not our eyes seen this before, and have not our ears heard this before?" she answers that truth sometimes comes from where it is least expected. Though the "Great Ones" may doubt that which is "pourest forth by a vessell that is altogether unlikely," the problem is not with the "liquor" spouting from an unlikely conduit, but with the obdurate refusal of a resistant audience to "lend your ears." Trapnel, however, knows better and insists that "the Lord hath accomplished his design in this work" that is "thy servant" (*Cry* Sig. $L1_v$/74). The truth she offers may not pour into the hearing of the unwilling, but she will nevertheless impart it to be taken up in "the bosom of them that have heard these beatings of thy Spices." Moving from a fluid metaphor that passes too quickly through the ears of the willfully deaf "Great Ones" to the more solid form of spice underscores the potentially greater staying power of the latter, at least for those who "have their senses open to feel the smell thereof" (*Cry* Sig. $L1_v$/74). The *synaesthesia* of a feeling smell may be unknowingly and even unfortunately mixed, but the metaphor brings the more tangible and durable sense of touch to a scent that might otherwise prove as ephemeral as the unreceived flowing liquor.[20]

Going on to depict herself as a "poor worm" who might nevertheless be "delivered from all Satanical delusions and evil beasts" with the assistance of prayer, she aspires thus to "sweetly solace her self in thy bosom among the still-waters, as upon the great Seas." Striking in its

[19] As Magro points out, "Trapnel's ecstatic prophesies and her conscious pronouncements," did not work to distinguish but "demystified the ideological interdependency of state and religious apparatuses." Pointing to her later work, where Trapnel proclaims that "one depends upon another, Rulers upon Clergie, and Clergie upon Rulers" (*Report and Plea* 21), Magro notes that she "boldly proclaimed the imminent inversion of the current social hierarchy" (421). What Magro does not specify is how the four horns she describes here likewise work to illustrate an interdependence upheld also in the *antimetabolic* form of the *Rulers/Clergie/Clergie/Rulers* that articulates and illustrates her later assertion.

[20] Like Donne, Trapnel understands that "knowledge of the soul, like all knowledge," as Stephen Pender puts it, "depends on the senses" in a world where the physical "indexes the metaphysical" ("Essaying the Body" 231–32).

sibilance, the image of the sea's still waters is also noteworthy in that the solace she finds comes with the ability not to mistake "the shining of a Glow-worm" for "the shining of the Sun," as too often happens in an age when "any thing is taken for holiness." Such "shells and outsides," she maintains, cannot withstand "the storm" that "is coming." The inner life of self-solace is not as complacent as the mere semblance of holiness the empty and inert shell may suggest. Unlike the "outsides," the inner "life of vision here is excellent, and precious, and glorious," Trapnel avers in a *polysyndeton* alluding to a beneficence expressed in a heaping-up of "ands" that could easily go on. All of this is brought to her by the power of "Vision," she exclaims, an inner sight so powerful "the body crumbles before it, and becomes weak." Reversing the effects of an illness that brought about her prophecies in the first place, sight brings the now-welcome effect of weakening a body suggestive in its crumbling. As she goes on to explain, "men are mistaken when they think that the great things of God will puff up." Appearances can mistake, and it is not the visible grandeur of puffery but, she assures her audience, a "self-denying," discernible "humility" that "shall make a difference between that which is not, and that which is" (*Cry* Sig. $L1_v$/74). Offering to the humble the "hope" Hobbes equates with "Assurance," Trapnel does so through the many appeals to imagination Hobbes also prescribes in persuading "that the help is near" ("Of Assurance" 56).

Fashioning in her own defence an ethos that persuades by contrast, Trapnel distances her language from that of a clerical pack mistaken in thinking "the great things of God will puff up." In a minister who promised to satisfy those who spoke against her yet, she later discovered, "hath reproached me and other friends that are of more worth then I," she finds a very empty rhetoric. "All these words," she concludes, "and many other more, amounted to just nothing; it was but Clergie-puff, which soon was gone like a puff of winde that is almost at an end, as soon as it riseth, and so was his fair speech to me" (*Report* Sig. $D2_r$/19). "Clergie-puff" is precisely the kind of rhetoric that Collins, Eliza, and Trapnel are able to transcend because they are not clergy but are divinely marked and sometimes empowered by affliction; as Eliza puts it in "The Support," "I dare not say, I am an ignorant woman, and unfit to write, for if thou wilt declare thy goodness, and thy mercy be weak and contemptible means, who can resist thy will" (75) or, as Collins writes in her "Verses on the twelvth Chapter of *Ecclesiastes*" (85–88), "they have no Scripture (I suppose) / Save what they wrest unto their own Perdicion" (lines 61–62). What she has that "they" do not is a spiritual understanding that comes also through the body: "the word with bower goes," she goes on in a reference to Hebrews 4.12,[21]

> Twixt Soul & Spirit by divine commission
> Twixt joynts and marow it doth penetrate,
> Seeing all secrets, heart can meditate.
> (lines 63–66)

Like Prideaux, whose *Sacred Eloquence* also draws on Hebrews in uniting the physical "joints and marrow" with the metaphysical "soul and spirit," the poet confirms the capacity of divine language to afflict both body and soul. For Collins as well, God's omniscience extends as deeply into the "joynts and marow" as it does the "Soul & Spirit," and Eliza and Trapnel equally confirm that the access to the Word demands a heightened awareness of the body.[22]

Hence the Word who is flesh brings another kind of suffering in his divine incarnation, what Richard Sibbes in his 1639 *Bowels opened, or, A discovery of the neere and deere love, union and communion betwixt Christ and the Church, and consequently betweixt Him and every believing soule* describes as the spiritual but equally welcome "sicknesse of love to Christ" (312). But Sibbes's metaphorical rendering also collapses distinctions between body and soul and, in keeping with a Trinity whose three parts are equally divine, suggests a conflation of wounder and healer not so different from the Hebrew God's. The interconnection of flesh and spirit in religious devotion is confirmed even in the visceral title of a work echoing Trapnel's claim to have "related what bowels of compassion from the Lord I found" (*Report* Sig. $E3_r$/29). Sibbes argues that one is fortunate enough to suffer such a sickness

> only if our love bee in such a degree, as it makes us sick of it, it makes us not to heare what wee heare, not to see, what wee see, not to regard what is

21 God's knowledge, the passage reads, is "piercing even to the dividing asunder of soul and spirit, and of the joints and marrow, and is a discerner of the thoughts and intents of the heart" (Heb. 4.12).

22 Hence these writers show themselves knowing participants in a larger, male-dominated discourse that, as Stephen Pender puts it, had long seen "physicians and philosophers argue for an intricate, intimate relationship between bodies and souls" that regarded the soul as "custodian of the body." Such a view, Pender explains, was predicated on a number of sources, including the "scripture" and "quotidian experience" on which these women writers explicitly draw as they evince their less explicit but perhaps equal awareness of sources Pender describes as "sophisticated conceptions of the interchange between matter and spirit" ("Subventing" 210). What Collins describes here is further suggestive of Richard Sugg's "smoke of the soul," the less than fully articulated answer to the frightening clarity of the Christian duality that encompassed a "material and perishable" body and an "immaterial and immortal" soul: the solution was the vague sense that "the body was united to the soul by means of the spirits" that, Sugg explains, "were a kind of fine vapour, steaming or smoking from the thinnest and most active part of the blood" (3). For Collins, it seems that the Word is the catalyst that enables the spirits connecting the soul to the "joynts and marrow."

> present: the soul is in a kind of extasie, it is carried so strongly and taken up with things of Heaven, it is deaded to other things, when our eyes are no more led with vanity, then if wee had none, and the flesh is so mortified, as if wee were dead men, by reason of the strength of our affections that runne another way to better things which are above ... Thus wee see it is in love. (312)

One cannot transcend what one does not know, and sometimes that knowledge comes to the faithful through the peculiar advantages of illness. Making room for the "reason of the strength of our affections," the suffering that sooner or later comes to all may in many ways be a great equalizer. Unlike the minister who promised to deliver but healed nothing, Collins, Eliza, and Trapnel find in affliction a rhetoric that, contrary to a blowhard emptiness of mere words, actually gets something done.

Finding a measure of empowerment in suffering that is never held apart from religion, Collins, Eliza, and Trapnel focus neither on illness nor on learned medicine, but their work is akin to that of male writers such as Donne at least insofar as their rhetorical purpose is to achieve solace. Unlike Donne and despite their many disclaimers to the contrary, however, the three women reveal a like intention to share their comfort in an intent more public than can be ascribed to the meditational and thus inherently private mode of Donne's *Devotions*. Through the affliction of illness and in their writing about it, Collins, Eliza, and Trapnel not only represent the advantages they find, but direct their understanding to an audience broader than the selves their writing serves also to fashion. In doing so, they also resist some widely asserted beliefs about women's rhetorical ability and appropriate behaviour. Attributing her affliction to a lie of omission and asserting her own healing ability over the physician's, Halkett addresses both, finding in illness the means of asserting her authority and proving herself innocent of a more grievous fault. Whether discovering through the afflicted body a corollary empowering of mind and spirit or, in Halkett's case, the means of fashioning an ethos appropriate to a woman of "religion and virtue" (32), all four women, like Donne, write from a devotion that also leaves them nothing to fear.

Unlike her Interregnum antecedents, Mary Astell finds in affliction more torment than advantage but, like Halkett, she explicitly takes up the topic of physicians. Included among the *Six Familiar Essays* published in 1696, her explicitly persuasive epistle does more to question physical suffering than accept it.[23] Writing in "An Essay of Sickness" to a friend "who

[23] Astell's persuasive eloquence as an essayist is now well established, and Christine Mason Sutherland's *The Eloquence of Mary Astell*, a thoughtful and expansive study of Astell's rhetoric and the thinking that informed it, has done much to retrieve her from intellectual obscurity. "Something of a

had been dangerously Ill," she also recognizes an affliciton brought about by the will of a God who sometimes "sees fit to lay severe pain or sickness either upon our selves" as well as "those who are dear to us" (Sig. $D4_r$–$D4_v$/ 39–40). Astell may also read affliction as evidence of a deity who is actually paying attention, but she does more to challenge than uphold what is articulated in Collins, Eliza, and Trapnel as well as some better-known works by their male counterparts. Contrary to what Taylor's *Rule and Exercises* asserts, physical suffering for Astell does not bring about the fallen world's equivalent of "Adams early morning in Paradise" (109). Rather than infusing the peace that might passeth understanding, illness does not ameliorate but, Astell insists, "multiplies all our other Grievances." Rendering the sufferer "incapable of pleasures," bodily affliction also affects an intellect dulled in sympathy with the body. Far from inspiring poetic production or prophesying, "the weakness of the body has such effect upon the mind," Astell maintains, "that it sinks under those troubles that would not move it at another time" (41–42). Acknowledging an interdependence of mind, body, and spirit that sees "our Judgment decaying with us," she finds only debilitation in illness. Though bodily affliction may inspire the imagination, it does so to adverse and not fruitful effect. Rather than impelling the intellect that otherwise "should fill the breast with well digested thoughts," illness displaces reason with "wild Chimera's of our own" so that we "startle every moment at Gyants of our own raising up" (42).

Like Donne, Astell specifically takes up the topic Collins, Eliza, and Trapnel overlook as she addresses the practice of medicine along with the miseries of illness. Uniting theory and practice, she points out that "the learned have been convinced by many years experience, that vapours mimick all other Diseases" (44) and upholds learned medicine's authority over the tenuous understanding of the sufferer. The deceptive nature of an illness that "raises the Vapours" (43) results in a patient who "not only obstructs the cure," she writes to her friend, but is also "ready to grasp at the least Discouragement." In the throes of what they will "represent more dangerous than it proves," sufferers will also take exception "if you question their understanding in the case" (44). The "Vapours" are, she explains,

> a Distemper which fills the Imagination with a thousand terrifying whimsies; and not only alters, but totally deprives us of our senses, and appears like a forerunner of Death to them that see, as well as they who feel, its most

celebrity in her own day" but later fallen from favour, Astell may have been, as Sutherland claims, "the most important woman rhetorician of her time" (xi–xvii).

> amazing symptoms; this sort of illness varies very often and baffles both them that prescribe, and them that apply the Remedies; and much less can they, who are overcome by the apprehensions of its fatal Consequences, give a just account of themselves; for it seizes so deeply upon their Intellects, that they read their doom in every sad look. (43)

Though Astell may here deny that "some humoral treatises seem to aim specifically at increasing their readers' sense of autonomy, offering greater knowledge and control of their own humoral makeup as a means of self-fashioning" (153), as Selleck proposes, she nevertheless implies a degree of patient autonomy, perhaps even agency, in an illness that "fills the Imagination." Rather than offering the greater knowledge and control Selleck identifies, however, Astell argues that the humours cannot be controlled, working as they do not only to adverse effect on the body but also impairing "Intellects" that can no longer read or even be read aright. Even writing consolation to the friend who likely feared for her life, Astell sees little advantage in the illness she describes. Those who "prescribe" and those who follow the learned physician and "apply the Remedies," she also suggests, are baffled. Impaired by "apprehensions" discernible in "every sad look," Astell's healers suffer a fear akin to that Donne reads in the countenance of his own physicians.

Astell nevertheless champions a male-dominated profession that may be sometimes helpless in the face of disease, but does have merits. What the "learned" have discovered through observation, she goes on to explain, is that those vapours "deceive" no one "so much as those that have 'em." In Astell's view, the patient is the least equipped to determine treatment or even to judge the nature or extent of the affliction. The Vapours that induce "melancholy will raise the Spleen in Sickness (and sometimes in Health) to such a height that they almost die daily in their belief." Unlike Donne, Halkett, and the Interregnum poets and prophesiers, Astell makes it clear that the illness she describes does not enable devotion or enhance religious understanding. On the contrary, those who "die daily" do so "not in the Apostle's meaning," as in Paul, by whose own faith "in Christ Jesus our Lord, I die daily" (1 Cor. 15.31) in perpetual regeneration of devotion. For Astell, the degenerating, metaphorical daily death of the afflicted applies even to the most devout, "for tho the best of Christians are as liable to this misfortune as any other," it has naught to do with devotion, she parenthetically confirms, "it being a defect in Nature not in Grace" (44). In the worst of cases, illness can diminish faith to the point of negation. Hence she urges her friend vigilant in maintaining her own, for "a disturbed Conscience is certainly the saddest Circumstance of a sick friend, and I heartily beseech God to keep me and all I am concerned in, from falling into it, that we may never have a distrust of our Salvation through Jesus Christ" (52–53).

Astell's peroration calls to a virtuous action that resists the many disadvantages of illness. Urging resistance against the coming "night of Affliction either in body or mind," Astell appeals to her reader to "let us make our calling and Election more sure" by preemptive preparation for what comes to all. Debilitating to the body and mind, illness necessarily afflicts also the soul to which they are integrally linked. Preparing for illness is therefore more important to Astell than coping with it, "for when we are declining in our healths, or clouded in our thoughts," she avers, we must at least be able to recognize "how unfit are we to Judge of, or to improve our Soul's Condition" (54). It is telling, however, that the damage she anticipates can be redressed with the language of persuasion, working as it does to prepare body and mind for the "night" of the soul. For Astell, the advantages of illness are found in its inevitability, an exigence that requires the careful reasoning of proper preparation. Astell thus signs off with apology for her own loquacious fault: "But I forget," she admits, "much reading may incommode you," and thereby compromise the intentions of one who writes only to "wish you all Health" (55).

Sounding much like Astell, clergyman Timothy Rogers is equally skeptical not only of the advantages others attach to illness, but also of those who profess to treat it. Writing "After his Recovery from a Sickness of near two years continuance," the title page tells us, his *Practical Discourses on Sickness & Recovery* (1691) focuses on illness's debilitating effects. Rather than enabling language as it does for Collins, Eliza, and Trapnel, illness for Rogers can remove the capacity even to utter what might facilitate healing. Indeed, he writes, "A Thousand things may hinder your having any Relief from Physitians: You may be so pained as not to be able to give them an account how you are, or what part is affected, or after what manner" (Sig. $D2_r$/35). From both a patient and a clerical perspective, Rogers knows what it is to be rendered silent. Losing not only the capacity for speech but also any potential to help the healing process, the mute patient limits access to medical knowledge that therefore remains "below the threshold of the visible and the expressible" (Foucault, Intro.). Denying the ability of medicine perhaps to do any good, Rogers defies the claims of physicians, who despite "all their Learned Art," face an "abundance of secret and violent disease into which they cannot penetrate" (Sig. D_v/34). Like Astell, Rogers warns of the dangers of misreading in the face of the silent and suffering. A patient may, for instance, "have several complicated illnesses, and what they prescribe for one, may be very prejudicial to another." Worse, the physician "may do it in haste, or by a wrong Judgment," make errors of carelessness, "which is very easie to fallible Men" he parenthetically acknowledges, and "take that for your Disease which really is not so" (Sig. $D2_v$/36).

For Rogers as much as Browne, the "little world" Donne describes as so "cunningly" made (Holy Sonnet 5, line 1) is not merely "a pleasant trope of rhetoric," but reveals in its complexity "a real truth therein" (Browne, *Religio* 24; part 1, sec. 34). The human microcosm presents as many mysteries, and, writes Rogers, "there are many things in this little World Man, that are to the most knowing as a *Terra Incognita*, and there may be a Thousand Diseases for with they want a name, and much more a Cure, and for which there is no Receipt in all the Dispensatories in the World" (Sig. D_v–$D2_r$/34–35). Rogers is willing to concede that "their Profession indeed is Learned," but insists that medicine need also acknowledge the limits of knowledge applicable to "all other Humane Sciences" likewise "full of imperfections." That this is so is verified by the impermanence of an art that yet looks to the far-off ancients for its authority, denying in the process "the Light which has broke out by the Discoveries and Inquiries of Latter Ages even as to many things in the very frame and contexture of Humane Bodies, which were not known before, shews the darkness and ignorance of former Ages, and when this has done its best, the next will its like see more." Anticipating a paradigm shift yet in the making, Rogers avers that, however much his age might believe it knows about "Humane Bodies" and their treatment, their "darkness and ignorance" will become readily apparent in the next. For Rogers, there is only one immutable truth, and it is not earthly: "Beware of leaving your dependence on God to put your trust in Men," he cautions, "And though it is commonly said every one is to be believed in his own Art, yet that belief very easily degenerates into presumption" (Sig. $D2_r$/35).

The mistaking dangers identified by Astell and Rogers come to the forefront in clergyman Richard Baxter's 1696 *Reliquiae Baxterianae*, whose first part, he reveals in the opening synopsis, was "written for the most part in 1664." In his posthumously published autobiography, Baxter writes of an illness relevant to his understanding of grace, recognizing with Halkett, Collins, Eliza, and Trapnel that "the Case of my *Body* had a great Operation upon my Soul." After suffering measles at seven and smallpox at fourteen, Baxter evidently developed "a violent Catarrh and Cough" that "continued about two years" to render him "much afraid of a Consumption" of the kind that was "then common in the Country" and was followed by "the Spitting of Blood" that "increased my fears." Taking the advice of "Sir *Henry Herbert*" to treat with "the Flower of Brimstone," his cough improved, but the prescribed therapy also "increased the acrimony of my Blood" (Sig. C_r/9). Subsequently diagnosed by "an unskillful Physician" who "perswaded me that I had a Hectick," he followed up in consultation with "an Aged and Experience Doctor," whose prescribed treatment for scurvy that "abundantly increased my bleeding at the Nose" by "half a Pint or a Pint a day" he followed for two years. Subsequently consulting "no less than Six and thirty Physicians" at whose direction he "us'd Druggs without number almost" and finally from "all Authors that I read" learning "that my Disease was incurable," he ultimately "forsook Doctors for the most part," though "when the urgency of a Symptom, or Pain" arose, would nevertheless be compelled "to seek some present ease." That he was "never overwhelm'd with real Melancholy" was the first of "two wonderful Mercies" he received "from God." The second was that his pain, "though daily and almost continual did not very much disable me from my Duty," but allowed him to "study, Preach, and Walk almost as well" (Sig. C_v/10) as if he had not been ill.

Further consultations with physician Theodore Mayerne (who tended Charles I), a three-week visit to the "*Tunbridge*-Waters," and written exchanges seeking counsel from physician George Bates (who tended Charles II) brought advice for similarly concurring courses of treatment that proved equally ineffective.[24] After trying what may have been all of the physicians' means at his disposal, Baxter finally hit upon his own four-part remedy for health, involving temperate eating, sweat-inducing exercise, the company of hot fires, and "beer as hot as my Throat will endure," which together with "on Herb inwardly taken" kept him in health at least to his current age of nearly seventy. Baxter concludes that "these are the Means which God hath used to draw out my days," and he writes his account of how "almost all Physick did me harm" to the benefit "of any Students that may be near the same Distempers" (Sig. $C2_r$/11). Though meriting a "brief Account," Baxter warns of his experience with medicine, "it is not a Matter worthy to be oft mentioned" (Sig. C_r/9).

[24] That Baxter "never escaped from doctors" and "was always asking their opinion despite his rejection of them" points to how difficult it was to find the "epistemological freedom" he sought; that "Baxter was fighting the doctors" throughout his memoir, Wear goes on, further attests to "how much power they had in his eyes and how necessary a diagnostic label was for Baxter to legitimate his disease" ("Puritan Perceptions" 93–94). Wear's observation attests to the extent to which medicine depended (and yet depends) on Foucault's signifying word as well as a medical context everywhere inflected by learned medicine's persuasive efforts.

What might otherwise be a very lengthy tale of a years-long experience with some two score of physicians is thus given necessary but only peripheral room in Baxter's story. What is most important for him is the wealth of evidence he possesses from his own experience, a heaping up of *exempla* so persuasive in their number they require little amplification and thus discount to a greater as well as more specific degree the merits of a profession Rogers is at least willing to acknowledge as learned. Baxter thus chooses experience over an authority whose bookish epistemology has, in his case, done much more harm than good. Denying the evidence before their very eyes, the physicians cannot do what "riding much in the Army" (Sig. C_v/10) and a regimen developed from the need to tend his own blood grants to this patient – an understanding of his body that easily surpasses that of learned medicine. Despite what may seem needless suffering at the hand of treatments mostly ineffectual and sometimes dangerous, because "the Soul is not *awaked* so much by *fear* and *care* to make resistance" (8), Baxter has gained from bodily affliction the benefits to mind and spirit brought about by apprehension and diligence. Also understanding "pain and illnesses not as medical entities but as the language that God used" (Wear, "Puritan Perceptions" 97), Baxter lends credence to a claim he makes from the patient's perspective, that "the Servants of God" are indeed the "men of *most knowledge*" (8).

Recognizing with Collins, Eliza, and Trapnel that illness is the language of God, it turns out that Baxter also shares the "Hypocondriack Melancholy" (Sig. C_v/10) akin to the "melancholy, by reason that the bloud faileth" Fonteyn ascribes uniquely to the female sex (Sig. $C3_r$/25). Baxter is not, however, the only writer to suggest that such disorders were not utterly exclusive to women. Aiming to mediate the new and orthodox in his 1667 *The Chymical Galenist,* George Castle explicitly challenges gendered notions of illness in his epistemology-bridging treatise. Acknowledging that "though the Disease called *Hysterica Passio,* be by almost all Authors treated of as only peculiar to Women, and proceeding only from the distemperature of the Womb," he claims to have discovered something quite different. Challenging the learned physicians' theory-privileging epistemology in averring the equal value of "Reason and Experience," Castle argues that women's medical history may not tell hysteria's whole story: "yet (as I have before observed) it may," he insists, "be very truly affirmed, That Men also are liable to most of the Symptoms of it, and that even in Women they are often caused when the Womb is not in the least concern'd in the guilt." This discrepancy in women, he concludes, is most likely attributable to "their more delicate constitution" (48) rather than the womb that, in views like Sadler's, is the undisputed and "evill" cause of multiple and varied maladies.

Though it remains unclear which disease caused the illnesses of Halkett, Collins, Eliza, and Trapnel or of Astell's friend, it is telling that Baxter's was, like theirs, treated through an understanding of the body that grew in conjunction with the awakening of the soul. Rather than overtly challenging the physicians, however, the women writers who do offer a patient's perspective present a view of illness that responds, for the most part, not to any described medical treatment but to their own attentiveness to matters devotional and spiritual in their varying accounts and uses of illness. Evincing a clear awareness of the nuanced ways their culture conceived of affliction and treatment as well as rhetorical norms of credible evidence and persuasive argument, women who wrote about illness and healing proved in many ways as rhetorically capable as the men whose texts aim in various ways to contain and control them. Far from being too easily confounded "with a more Rhetoricall discourse" as Sadler would have it ("The Epistle Dedicatory" n. pag.), that some women afflicted by illness proved themselves full and knowing participants in the rhetoric of learned medicine is discernible also in their collective tendency to occlude the physician as much as the physician-authored treatises that ignore, subject, or malign the patients who are their very raison d'être.

CHAPTER 5

"Hard Words and Rhetoricall Phrases"
Women and Learned Medicine

In "The Epistle Dedicatory," physician John Sadler directly addresses the women readers of his 1636 *The Sick Womans Private Looking-Glasse* (1636). Deigning to share his medical knowledge, Sadler lets his feminine audience know that he has in their interest "stooped to your capacities in omitting hard words and Rhetoricall phrases" and thereby avoided the "more Rhetoricall discourse" that is clearly beyond their reach (n. pag.).[1] In his 1656 epistle "To the Reader," however, Richard Bunworth professes instead to be "somewhat indulgent to their modesty" in avoiding "all obscenity," and to accommodate women's lesser "capacity in writing in our mother tongue." Thus doing "reall service to the female sex," Bunworth's *The Doctresse* offers specific directions for how the knowledge proffered from "continuall experience" might fulfill its aim "to informe the ignorant." The less-than-learned user must, the author advises, peruse the book "twice over," reading it "first cursorily, that thou maist have a generall conceit of the thing I do intend" and only "then with some observation, that thou maist so digest it" (n. pag.). Content whose proper perusal requires instruction and effort for women is, Bunworth also makes clear, for "the learned" a collection of mere "hints" accessible with corresponding ease. Showing little faith in the feminine reader's ability to comprehend readily even a text addressed specifically "to their capacity," Sadler and Bunworth assert women ill equipped to engage the discourse of learned medicine even as they profess an intent to provide helpful instruction to their sex.

Protecting the persuasive art that proved key to the physicians' success and asserting women ill equipped to negotiate "Rhetoricall discourse," books like Sadler's and Bunworth's exclude as much as include the audience

[1] Curiously, "The Epistle Dedicatory" is followed by two additional paratexts in Latin. It is debatable whether Sadler presumed his readers accomplished enough to know Latin, and his previous comments are therefore meant in jest, or whether he assumed his female audience would be unable to read the texts, and his choice therefore aims to prove his point. Given the context, however, he likely meant to remind women of their intellectual inferiority.

they simultaneously address and alienate. As they take particular aim at the "petticoat" doctors and midwives whose practice they increasingly claimed, however, the physicians may protest too much.[2] Their insistence in defining a specialized discourse that, even in the vernacular, was beyond the grasp of the simpler sex may, in fact, imply something quite different from the female inadequacy they insist upon. Suggested by the physicians' proprietary exclusion of women altogether or, as in the case of Sadler and Bunworth, their questioning of women's capacity to engage a discourse too difficult even its simplest form, it may be that women's persuasive potential presented as great a challenge to the physicians' proclaimed dominion as their culturally understood capacity for healing. Contrary to what the physicians' insinuations and assertions suggest, a lack of formal education as well as numerous injunctions against their public speech do not also mean that women did not actively and knowingly participate in rhetorical culture, and, as we have seen, some proved as capable of taking up the discourse Sadler and Bunworth avoid as others were in practising the profession denied.[3]

Writing from the healer's perspective, poet Anne Bradstreet, midwife Jane Sharp, and physician Jane Barker offer three very different examples

[2] The kind of medical work women undertook often varied by class but, Patricia Crawford notes, "paid and unpaid" women "at all levels of society" participated (66). Accomplished healers, women may have provided what Margaret Pelling proposes was "the most important stratum of care in Jacobean England" ("Trade or Profession" 250). Summarizing Ronald Sawyer's analysis of Bedfordshire case records in "Patients, Healers, and Disease in the Southeast Midlands, 1597–1634" (University of Wisconsin-Madison PhD thesis, 1986), Pelling points out that women performed a critical role in early modern medicine even as unofficial practitioners as they assumed primary responsibility in caring for the poor, tending to illness in the home, treating wounded soldiers, and delivering babies, thus countering William Kerwin's assertion that late sixteenth-century women were "still doing significant medical work," but the seventeenth century saw them "gradually driven into the shadows" (95). The extent of women's knowledge and practice, A. S. Weber argues, further challenges the assumption that there was "a dichotomy between male and female medical knowledge" (375). As Pelling and Webster note, "twenty-nine female practitioners" were "prosecuted by the college of Physicians between 1550 and 1600," and they "almost certainly represent only a fraction of the women practitioners," of whom "many specialized primarily in the medical problems of women and children." Moreover, they argue, "it is likely that nurses as well as midwives were apt to trespass into medical practice" (186–87). The rise of the "man-midwife," and the appropriation of midwifery into a male-dominated obstetrics and gynecology have been well documented, most especially by Monica Green in *Making Women's Medicine Masculine*. That women had long participated in European medicine, some as physicians and surgeons trained by husbands or fathers, is also well documented by historian Leigh Whaley in *Women and the Practice of Medical Care in Early Modern Europe, 1400–1800*.

[3] Healers of every kind may have participated in shaping the discourse the physicians sought to protect. "All practitioners," as Harley argues, "from university graduates to village wise women, had to provide explanations that satisfied those who consulted them" and, in its shared aim to persuade prospective or existing patients as well as counterparts and rivals, all "medical writing can profitably be seen as competition for the control of meaning" ("Social Construction" 414–15).

that, taken together, suggest something of the extent to which women drew their own authorial and medical authority from the language of learned medicine, and that they did so while sometimes also resisting the injunctions and insinuations of its hegemonic and exclusionary rhetoric.[4] That all three took up medical topics but lived and worked in very different circumstances and wrote in varying genres attests as well to medical knowledge and practices that were not homogeneous but as varied as those of their male counterparts. Illustrating the "subtle division of labour" Hilary Rose associates with "the different lives of women in the middling classes, and the aristocratic women" as well as distinctions associated with professional and lay, their example also suggests that the well-educated women who more often were aristocratically connected were also more closely acquainted with the knowledge of learned medicine, while those "in the middling classes," as Rose proposes, "tended to be stronger on empirical knowledge" (xiv). Though it is true that Sharp is clearly of the middling class while the extent of Bradstreet's and Barker's educations aligns them more closely with the upper, all three can be seen to draw on the rhetoric of learned medicine in fashioning their own authority. Confirming their understanding of a profession epistemologically and practically dependent on the art of persuasion as they inscribe their inclusion within it, Bradstreet, Sharp, and Barker thus illustrate women's active and varied engagement in its discourse as they confirm their understanding of healing knowledge and practice.

As she engages the discourse of learned medicine in her 1650 collection *The Tenth Muse*, New England poet Anne Bradstreet proves intent on her own self-fashioning.[5] In the ambitious and wide-ranging quaternions that, in addition to the elements and seasons, consider the nature of the four humours as well as childhood, youth, middle, and old ages and the various ailments that go with them, however, Bradstreet fashions a judicious and credible ethos not by invoking the evidence of experience or the proof

[4] Royal Society interloper Margaret Cavendish is another mid-century woman who explicitly engaged seventeenth-century medical discourse. As Jacqueline Broad explains, Cavendish was especially interested in van Helmont, the disciple of Paracelsus, who called "for a complete overthrow of traditional medicine" (50). Her interest did not result in unequivocal endorsement, however: in her *Worlds Olio* of 1655, Cavendish "clearly supports Galen's theory of the humors" even though her *Philosophical Letters* "supports van Helmont's new ontological conception of disease" as external to the patient (51).

[5] Initially published in London by her brother-in-law, who purportedly took the manuscript to England without the author's knowledge, the volume's lengthy works along with some shorter were republished posthumously in Boston as *Several Poems* (1678). My focus is on the original 1650 collection.

of pious devotion. Though likely a domestic healer herself in a community that lacked medical professionals but upheld the interdependence of "spiritual means" and "material agents" that, Norman Gevitz points out, also meant "ministers and health care practitioners ideally played complementary roles" (10), Bradstreet shows little interest in taking the part of the physician–clerics or in asserting her place among those who actually practised healing. Rather than the practical and religious emphases we might expect from a future mother of eight who lived in a deeply religious and medically underserved colony, Bradstreet emphasizes not a divinely ordained mandate to heal nor the healing power of the Word; nor does she champion women's practical knowledge. Focusing instead on the texts and tenets of learned medicine, Bradstreet's rhetoric most clearly aligns with that of the elite practitioners who were the physician–clerics' and the woman healers' oft-professed opposition, fashioning in her quaternions an ethos that stands not in competition but in concert with that of the male-constructed authority the physicians represented and defended.[6]

Bradstreet's intellectual sympathy with learned medicine makes itself known also in style and substance that stand out, Anne Hildebrand observes, as "elaborate in a way Anne Bradstreet never attempted again" (117).[7] The singularity of the quaternions may, of course, have much to do with Bradstreet's gradual adaptation to life in colonial New England, where "the real overseer of practitioners' activities was the community" (Gevitz

[6] Accordingly, Bradstreet's devotional work does not conflate but upholds the distinction of religious and medical professions. Modelled after the French protestant DuBartas, whose *Divine Weekes and Workes* was translated by Joshua Sylvester and published in 1605, Bradstreet's quaternions inevitably participate in a convention of "Puritan sermons and writings" that "embraced the will of God as revealed in nature and the experience of individual lives" (365) as Virginia Brackett claims, and they also reiterate the tenets of original sin and redemption. At times as well, Bradstreet takes up a mode more meditative than doctrinal. Apostrophizing to her dead father the hope that "my Fathers God, be God of me and mine" (Sig. O5v/218) and offering up a dialogue after Paul (Gal. 5.16–26) in the much-lauded lyric "The Flesh and the Spirit," for example, Bradstreet ventures into a genre well known in the work of male writers like Donne and explored in the meditations of women poets like Collins and Eliza. Even so, Bradstreet tends to separate the medical from the devotional and, though *The Tenth Muse* has been criticized for the perceived limitations of what Elizabeth Wade White once described as the "ornate du Bartian shackles" of the male poet's *Divine Weekes and Workes* (361), it is telling that religion is not the focus of verse written in emulation of the much-admired hexameron. Following DuBartas's formal and generic lead while displaying her own knowledge of the texts and tenets of learned medicine may, in fact, have endowed Bradstreet with a voice more liberated than constrained by imitative exercise.

[7] Bradstreet's assertions of humility and unworthiness in "To her most Honoured Father Thomas Dudley" suggest an aim to distinguish her "meanly clad" (line 11) output from that of the opposite sex, yet her claims to medical knowledge and her demonstrable understanding of how professional authority is wrought by language artfully used suggest something quite different. Bradstreet's verse may be as "highly argumentative" (361) as White complains, but it is telling of the critic's gendered expectations that it is therefore perceived as more deserving of dismissal than recognition.

12), and women necessarily assumed roles more practical than speculative.[8] It is well known that Bradstreet initially resisted conforming to communal expectations but seems to have become more acquiescent as the years passed. The marked generic and substantive changes from Bradstreet's early, learned verse to her later domestic poetry certainly suggest as much, the latter compelling critics to emphasize her brand of "sentimental poetics" as one that "reimagined the public community through a domestic lens" (Van Engen 47).[9] The difference so notable from her early work to late may, however, also have much to do with Bradstreet's "dexterity in manipulating logic and rhetoric" (Eberwein 20) applied to a growing recognition that she needed to fashion an ethos more conventionally suited to a colony that saw the 1638 banishment and subsequent slaying of "the courageously opinionated" healer and heretic Anne Hutchinson (White 363).[10]

Bradstreet nevertheless denies her obvious command of the art that served also to fashion the learned physician, confirming to readers early on that from her "no rhet'ric we expect" ("The Prologue" line 15).[11] In her later lament of "Four Monarchies," Bradstreet further maintains that

[8] As Jean Marie Lutes reminds us, "Caring for bodies in seventeenth-century New England was in many ways a female calling: the vast majority of women gave birth with the aid of other women, not men, and the burden of keeping children healthy fell primarily on women, many of whom could not have found a male doctor to call had they wanted to consult one" (310).

[9] Abram van Engen also notes that, although earlier criticism divided Bradstreet's corpus into "public and private strains," later critics identified both "domestic tropes and political concerns" throughout, while more recent readers suggest that "the public/private dichotomy in her poetry is both misleading and obsolete." Van Engen proposes that such readings "should still be tempered by the general shift in style and subject matter" (52). Regardless, it is ironic that the later, shorter poems written primarily to Bradstreet's family have garnered the most attention; as Eileen Margerum argues, it was the earlier "long formal poems" penned "according to age-old formulae" that Bradstreet most likely "intended as her bid for immortality" (158). That White's tercentary appraisal of Bradstreet apologizes for her earlier verse's "stilted and highly argumentative manner" while championing the glimmer of "grave and compassionated poetic image" more representative of the later work notable for its "maturity and a more personal approach" (361) says more about changing taste than Bradstreet's eloquence.

[10] Jeannine Hensley argues that the republished works appearing in 1678 as *Several Poems* "must contain more nearly the form in which she intended her work to appear" (xxxvii). Conversely, it may be that the earlier forms corresponded more closely with intentions later occluded out of self-protective necessity.

[11] As Patricia Pender has recently argued, critics have focused on Bradstreet's prefatory poem to the extent that it has become "representative of Bradstreet's poetic output," and thus "fails to do justice" to a poetic career spanning three decades and including some highly technical and demanding verse. Rather than accurately representing Bradsteet's ability or genuine ambition, Pender suggests, such an emphasis "coincides with and reinforces" our own desire to read through preconceived notions of gender that include "prevailing understandings of the early modern woman writer's fate at the hand of patriarchal oppression" (158). Like Pender, I aim to consider not how women were excluded – or excluded themselves – from the dominant discourses of their day, but the ways in which they engaged the culture in which they lived and wrote.

"I Rhetorick want to pour out execration" (Sig. G5$_r$/105) as she defers to Philip Sidney and "the spels that in his Rhetorick lurks" (Sig. N6$_r$/203). Linking her verse with his nevertheless, Bradstreet offers a gesture of modesty that is for both sexes as "conventional and obligatory" as Eileen Margerum suggests (159). Bradstreet is clearly an accomplished poet and rhetor, and her work may also be as performative as Sidney's.[12] That her speaking subject "Blood" has neither the "will nor art" for "acting" the "physician," "philosopher," or "anatomist" (Sig. C6$_v$–C7$_r$/28–29, lines 37–39) seems no less a gesture in a collection made up of multiple speaking voices equally intent on displaying the author's knowledge.[13] Bradstreet's misgivings may be voiced in the recognition that "Sweet Parnassus, I dote too much on thee" (Sig. B5$_v$/10, line 174), but expressed reticence does not prevent an address to "Ye *Galenists*" who "cure your patients" and "fill your purse with pence" by means of a feminized Earth who provides the "drugs that come from thence" (Sig. B6$_r$/11, lines 193–94).

More intent on displaying her knowledge of Galenic medicine, most notably in "Of the Four Humours in Man's Constitution," than in criticizing medical practice, Bradstreet makes clear her epistemological correspondence with the physicians, not least in proceeding from the premise that "male bodies are hotter than female bodies" (Lutes 315).[14] Bradstreet's verse also evinces her understanding of epistemologies that differ both in theory and in application through a speaking "Fire" that asserts her equal need among "Ye Paracelsians," who "in vain's your skill / In chemistry, unless I help you still," as well as the alchemical "philosophers," who "if e'er you made / A transmutation, it was through mine aid" ("Fire" lines 54–57). Even as she recognizes interdisciplinary interdependence, however, the poet upholds professional distinctions to which the unversed and uninitiated can lay no justifiable claim. The titular "Blood" may claim no desire

[12] Carrie Galloway Blackstock argues that Bradstreet the poet "maintains over time a multiple sense of self," but Bradstreet the woman "avoids having to reconcile facets of herself that were simply not reconcilable for a Puritan" (238).

[13] Margerum observes a criticial tendency to "see the strained tone and apologetic language" of "public poems" that include the quaternions as evincing Bradstreet's "insecurity in the traditionally male role of public poet" upheld in contrast with "the confident voice and absence of apologies in the private poems" her later work is thought to represent. Such a reading, however, overlooks the rhetorical *exigence* Bradstreet addresses as a woman writing and, as Margerum puts it, leads to interpretations "based on the Romantic idea that the poet must mean what she says" (152). Not only do such readings seem rather naïve, they also overlook Bradstreet's considerable skill as a rhetor.

[14] Rebecca J. Tannenbaum points out that "medicine was not the exclusive domain of elite professionals in British North America." Arguing that "in seventeenth-century England and its colonies, domestic medicine did not differ much from learned," Tannenbaum concludes that "this situation was amplified by the scarcity of elite practitioners" in colonial New England (3).

"to play Philosopher" and "no list" to act as "phisician, nor Anatomist" (Sig. C6$_v$/28, lines 237–38), but the profession of "Water" to lack "wondering Aristotles wit" (Sig. B7$_r$/15, line 341) cannot deny the rhetorical art so integral to learned medicine. Author of the cold and wet that defines "The fleg" constitution (Sig. B8$_v$/16, line 356), Water may claim, "Nor will I speake of waters made by Art" but nevertheless extols how they can "to life, restore a fainting heart." Extending the *paralepsis*, "nor fruitfull dewes, nor drops from weeping eyes," Water invokes an effect distinctly rhetorical in that "which pitty moves, and oft deceives the wise." The invocation of pathos she professes neither to address, but goes on to do so in the tears "Nor yet of Salt, and Sugar, sweet and smart" that "when we list, to water we convert," (Sig. B8$_v$/16, lines 342–47) as her own rhetoric shows something quite different from what it tells.

As Bradstreet's speaking "Melancholy" confirms, "wisdome 'tis, my wisdom to conceale" (Sig. D2$_v$/36, line 478). Asserting the difference between inward reality and outward appearance, the Melancholy of Galenic cause acknowledges the importance of language to fashioning and protecting learned medicine's truth. Over the black humour, however, authority is not easily won. Melancholy is "unto diseases not inclin'd" as her companion "sisters," and therefore "Nor cold, nor hot, Ague, nor Plurisie; / Nor Cough, nor Quinsie, nor the burning Feavor" does Melancholy "feel to act his fierce indeavour" (Sig. D2$_v$/36, lines 479–81). Confirming a power akin to that Bunworth and others associate with fear's effect on the body, Melancholy admits, "My sicknesse cheifly [sic] in conceit doth lye," thus "what I imagine, that's my malady" (Sig. D2$_v$/36, lines 482–83). The poet may assert that "art can doe much" to redeem the weak, but she also recognizes the maxim "most sure," that "a weake or wounded brain admits no cure" ("The Prologue" Sig. B2$_v$/4, lines 25–26). As her sister "Choler" says, she is "peevish, Male-content" and "musing," hence "by misprisions, like to loose her wits" (Sig. C4$_r$/23, lines 73–74). Difficult to read and subject to misinterpretation, Melancholy cannot be wholly or confidently controlled by the language that creates and subjects. Bradstreet's understanding of the importance of artful persuasion to Galenic theory and practice is by no means simple or consistent but, like the rhetoric of the learned physicians, complex and sometimes contradictory.

Over the whole of Bradstreet's corpus, however, her readers most often overlook the poet's nuanced engagement with learned discourse, choosing instead to focus on the woman who is also a wife, mother, daughter, and puritan. Certainly, Bradstreet's domestic and family-centred contributions later included in what has become the definitive version of her work have done much to encourage the critical emphasis on the poet as first and foremost a woman. Even so, "Bradstreet's poetic voice," as Lutes points out, may reiterate larger cultural beliefs that confirm a "Puritan mistrust of the flesh," but it is equally true that the poet "does not connect the myriad fleshly problems to female weakness" (321). Rather than specifically feminine, the poetic voice Lutes describes is also distinctly rhetorical and, though Bradstreet may apologize for its shortcomings, Margerum is right to observe that "she never uses her sex as an excuse for writing poor poetry" (157). In much the same way as she resists ascribing general notions of spiritual, bodily, or authorial weakness to the specifically feminine, choosing instead to engage what was male-authored and authorized, so Bradstreet fashions a self who understands and participates in a discourse that worked hard to keep interlopers out. The author of "The Prologue" may recommend that we "let Greeks be Greeks, and Women what they are" and confirm that it is "but vaine, unjustly to wage war" against the men who "have precedency, and still excel," but her work makes it difficult to accept as sincere the corollary assertion that "men can doe best, and Women know it well" (Sig. $B2_v/4$, lines 39–42). Attesting more to Bradstreet's rhetorical awareness than her lesser ability, the poet acknowledges male "preheminence," but does so in clearing the way to ask her audience yet to "grant some small acknowledgement of ours" (Sig. $B2_v/4$, lines 43–44). Suggesting an author not always interested in distinguishing herself from the opposite sex, Bradstreet's rhetoric works to fashion a learned authority not exclusive to men, and the ambitiousness and range of her quaternions suggest a poet whose rhetoric sought something more than the "small acknowledgement" she claims.

Making no pretenses of feminine modesty, *The Midwives Book* follows the physicians in asserting its authority from the very beginning. Announcing its author as "Mrs. Jane Sharp Practitioner in the Art of Midwifry above thirty years" (Sig. $A3_r$), the book's frontispiece suggests a text as intent on delineating and defending the bounds of learned medicine as offering medical guidance. Asserting who has the right and authority to practise midwifery, early modern manuals like Sharp's are thus as intensely rhetorical as Eve Keller proposes, engaging as they do "in the on-going debates about gender" while vying for "control of the birthing room" and "the human body" (102).[15] What Keller does not point out, however, is that the

[15] Though scholars have in recent decades identified the seventeenth century as a watershed moment in the history of women's medicine, one that saw the practice of obstetrics and gynecology finally taken over by men in the eighteenth, Monica Green instead posits that women "did not have anything like a *monopoly* over the production of knowledge on or care of the female body," and male

debate in which Sharp is so invested focuses as much on the language used as it does on using it for persuasive ends. Opening with a challenge to the physicians' hegemonic allegiance to Greek and Latin, Sharp's introduction draws a clear line between learned epistemologies and effective practice. Insisting that "it is not hard words that perform the work," Sharp argues that the physicians' linguistic gatekeeping is as unhelpful as it is transparent, a self-protective convention that may aim to uphold but cannot preserve their professionalizing mystique: "as if," she scoffs, "none understood the Art that cannot understand Greek."[16] Not only do the "hard words" of which the physicians are so fond fail to accomplish anything in and of themselves, given that they "are but the shell" of understanding, their inaccessibility can also cause figurative harm to the extent "that we ofttimes break our Teeth with them to come at the kernel" of the knowledge they fail or refuse to impart. Unnecessarily obfuscating at best and damaging at worst, the physicians' adherence to ancient language negates any aim to do good.

The figurative soon becomes literal, however, the metaphor enacted through a deliberately inaccessible discourse that not only impedes effective and efficient practice but violates the medical precept to do no harm. As Sharp goes on to explain, by metaphorical teeth "I mean our brains," which struggle "to know what is the meaning of them" though "to have the same in our mother tongue would save us a great deal of needless labour" (Sig. $B2_r$–$B2_v$/3–4). For Sharp, the physicians' language prevents ready access to medical knowledge, inhibiting rather than enabling the ethical mandate to provide care.[17] Bringing together the abstracted theory

physicians had always been involved in all aspects of women's heath care. "Far from being a 'modern' transformation," Green argues, "the masculinization of women's medicine is instead a fundamental feaure of western medicine down to its medieval roots" (ix). Green further suggests that the conflation of obstetrics and gynecology is a modern one, and that the two had long been separated, with women attending non-complicated births and men tending to difficult births as well as regular gynecological practice; hence the narrative is really "about the take-over of midwifery" (x).

16 Sharp lived and worked in an especially exclusionary medical context, given that elsewhere "the medical Renaissance came largely at second-hand through the dissemination of vernacular medical texts that handed down what were often diluted versions of Galenic teaching," but "the one great exception was the London College of Physicians, which expected its members to know the Latin texts of Galen and Hippocrates" (Wear, *Knowledge and Practice* 36). Hence it was somewhat more difficult for women than on the continent, where, Bridgette Sheridan notes, surgeons and midwives incorporated available medical theory "into their practices and, in some cases, into their own medical writing," and were thus "able to challenge the notion that physicians were the only 'learned practitioners'" (239).

17 Bicks reads the passage in light of Sadler's injunction, noting that "certain physicians like John Sadler imagined that they had 'stooped to your [women's] capacities' in avoiding hard words and Rhetoricall phrases" (Dedicatory Epistle), while "Sharp instead looks down on those learned men who insist on basing their knowledge in 'hard words' instead of hard work" (20).

the physicians' discourse withholds with the worldly experience their profession so often disdains, Sharp argues that the midwife's knowledge by contrast "must be twofold," encompassing both the "Speculative" and the "Practical" that reciprocally inform the work of the competent professional who need be well versed in both. "She that wants the knowledge of Speculation," Sharp argues, "is like to one that is blind or wants her sight," and "she that wants the Practice, is like one that is lame and wants her legs." Closing the analogy with the suggestively *antimetabolic isocolon* that "the lame may see but they cannot walk, the blind may walk but they cannot see" (Sig. $B1_v$/2), Sharp offers a mirrored and balanced form further underscoring the necessity of uniting an ever-reciprocal theory and practice. Beginning by "figuring herself as the gold standard of her profession" (5), as Caroline Bicks puts it, in contrast to those who do not comprehend the theoretical part of an "Art" dependent also the oppositional "authority of experience" (101) Keller identifies, Sharp opposes the persistently theoretical orientation advocated even by those physicians who acknowledge the importance of experience. Professing an intention more focused on medical need than professional mystique, her words confirm Keller's belief that the "resistance" of Sharp's text "to the Galenic system suggests that, rhetorically, it works to destabilize all male-constructed medical authority, whether ancient or modern, practical or theoretic" (108). In this and other ways, the exigence Sharp addresses demands a sustained challenge to the exclusionary, hegemonic discourse of the learned physicians.

At the same time, however, readings like Bicks's, which offers an extensive analysis of Sharp's "rhetorical revisions" as they disrupt the tropes of learned medicine (5), may miss the mark as much as Keller's in occluding the extent to which Sharp's self-fashioning aligns with the physicians'. Though discernible throughout, the persistently professionalizing bent of Sharp's text may be most salient at the beginning. Appealing to the "Sisters" of the prefatory epistle "To the Midwives of England," Sharp sounds very much like Cotta, Hart, or Primrose as she claims to have "often sate down sad in the Consideration of the many Miseries Women endure in the Hands of unskilful Midwives." Women suffer, Sharp maintains, because of those "many professing the Art (without any skill in Anatomy, which is the Principal part effectually necessary for a Midwife)" and thereby act only for "Lucres sake" (Sig. $A5_r$). Fashioning an ethos more altruistic and learned than her unqualified competition, she predicates her authority on the "Art" claimed also by the physicians, for she has studied the requisite anatomy "at Great Cost in Translation for all Books" (Sig. $A5_r$). Though acquired in the vernacular, Sharp lays claim to the knowledge of a profession whose persistent and self-protective adherence to ancient languages she also derides.

For Sharp, textual authority works in tandem with that she has accrued from "my own Experience." Like the physicians who make similar assertions, Sharp does not privilege experience over learning, but suggests the primacy of the latter in facilitating a practical understanding that remains inaccessible to those who do not also command at least some of the physicians' specialized knowledge. Hence Sharp fashions an ethos akin to Bradstreet's in positioning herself in league with the gatekeeping physicians while also contrasting her own expertise with the lack of those "unskilful Midwives." Sharp thus follows the physicians in claiming place over against those guided by experience alone. Like the physicians as well, she also laments those non-practitioners who might presume to intervene in or assume a role in patient care. Sounding much like Andrew Boorde, Sharp maintains that she "never could endure that preposterous way that most persons observe to the destruction of their Friends," an assertion offered with the example of patients provoked to eat when "fasting is the better Doctor" (Sig. $G5_r$/89). Sharp's self-fashioning thus works to champion knowledge superior to that of well-intentioned but misguided family and friends as well as that of less accomplished practitioners, implying if not forthrightly stating that not only her midwiferly competition but all members of a patient's household would do well to defer to her authority and, as Boorde would have it, therefore let "everie person be tendable about them, and do as they shall command them" ("A Preamble to sicke men and to those that bee wounded" n. pag.).

Like the physicians and the physician–clerics, Sharp claims a divinely ordained mandate to heal. Citing the Hebrew women's refusal to follow the Egyptian ruler's directive to slay all male children, she points out that "God dealt well with the Midwives" and, though neither Exodus 1.21 nor *The Midwives Book* specifies the nature of the "Houses" God "made them" in return (Sig. $B1_v$), both refer to a space granted to midwives alone. Whether literal or metaphorical, the scriptural example aligns with learned invocations of divine authority in construing communities of practice akin to the figurings of learned medicine. Holding allegiance to the qualitative discourse of an abstract epistemology, Wear notes, even late-century medical writing bears the discursive traces of an earlier age. Its ongoing reliance on "analogy and metaphor" in particular, Wear explains, indicates that the physicians' rhetoric may have been more nominally than actually transformed by shifting medical paradigms ("Continuity" 300). Sharp's reliance on the figurative thus suggests a discourse that in style as well as substance is as much in concert with as opposed to that of learned medicine. If Wear is right to suggest "that the empiric was a bit of a rationalist and vice versa" ("Continuity" 304) in a profession where unity was more the norm than the exception, then Sharp fully engages a discourse that, sometimes in spite of itself, relies on conventions only thought to be aligned with radically opposed epistemologies and practices.[18] Confirming continuity as it enacts union, Sharp's discourse represents the subjective, qualititative rhetoric Wear sees as erroneously ascribed to the physicians' past as well as the more objective, quantitative mode propounded by the empirics.

The Midwives Book thus bears discursive as well as substantive witness to the continuity and union Wear describes. Able to present in great detail the specifics of, for example, the circulatory system and the male and female reproductive organs, Sharp also evinces the "ability to tell the story from the seen (the effects) to the unseen (the causes)" that, according to Wear, "was from Greek times and up to and beyond the seventeenth century, the mark of the rational (and expensive) physician". Displaying a like "knowledge of causes" that distinguished the learned physician "from the crowd of empirics and quacks" ("Continuity" 297), the discursive traces Wear associates with learned medicine may also represent the most rhetorically distinctive characteristics of a text replete with analogy and metaphor. Acknowledging the extent to which *The Midwives Book* confirms "the disruptive potential of Sharp's rhetorical turn" (2–3), which Bicks claims on behalf of the book's figurative renderings, demands simultaneous recognition of Sharp's collusion with male authority in a way that facilitates the fashioning of her own.

Exemplifying the virtue of *enargeia* that renders description accessible and memorable, Sharp's richly figurative language happily coexists with a discourse marked by the literal, clinical description associated with an empiricist epistemology only thought to be incompatible. Sometimes those figures are familiar, as in her metaphorical description of the male "yard" as a plow, styling as she does the "man in the act of procreation" as the "agent and tiller and sower of the Ground" and his partner as "the Patient or Ground to be tilled" (Sig. $D1_r$/33), or the even more manly sword of a "French man" she heard "complain sadly" of a vagina once "no

[18] Sharp thus lends credence to Wear's claim that the inroads claimed by the seventeenth century's "new medicine" may overlook a "long view" ("Continuity" 300) suggesting more continuity than change in medical practice that remained strongly Galenic for another century or more. Churchill posits a similar finding over a longer period, discovering "far more continuity than change within the practice of British medicine during the period of 1590 to 1740" in a context that "promoted an emphasis on practitioner expertise and authority, especially amongst 'learned' physicians" (232–33).

bigger nor wider than would fit his turn" but now "grown as a Sack," the complaint of a man nevertheless also willing to recognize that "perhaps the fault was not the womans but his own, his weapon shrunk and was grown too little for the scabbard" (Sig. $E3_r$/53). At other times, however, Sharp's ability to "tell the story from the seen," the discursive mode Wear associates with the classical tradition of the physicians, is most effective in rendering the familiar strange, as when she describes the movement of male ejaculate from the "stones" to the "yard" as akin to the seeping migration of "quicksilver through a piece of leather" (Sig. $C1_r$/17).

In keeping with what Bicks sees as woman-centred "rhetorical revisions" (5), the *enargeia* of Sharp's bringing-before-the-eyes may be most readily on display in descriptions of the female genitalia with which her midwifery and her sex made her intimately familiar. Describing the nature and function of the *labia minor*, or what she calls "the wings that appear when the Lips are parted," Sharp presents a notably vivid passage replete with analogy and metaphor alongside the literal description associated with empiricism's quantitative leanings. Made of marginally figurative "soft spongy flesh" that literally entails "the doubling of the skin," the metaphorical wings are likened to "a Cocks Comb" in function, aiming as they do "to defend the Matrix from outward violence, and serve to the orifice of the neck of the womb" in a way analogous to the protection offered by the foreskin "to a mans Yard," and functioning to "shut the cleft with lips as it were, and preserve the womb from cold air and all injuries." Not merely defensive, however, "these wings besides the great pleasure they give women in Copulation" also "direct the Urine through the large passage" in utilitarian purpose analogous to the space that lies "between two walls" and is therefore also "like a Tunnel." Invoking the auditory as well as the visual, Sharp goes on to describe how the urine "runs forth in a broad stream and a hissng [sic] noise" deft in directing a flow that stays on course and "not so much as wetting the wings of the Lap as it goes along." Hence, she concludes in classical terms, "these wings are called Nymphs, because they joyn to the passage of the Urine, and the neck of the womb, out of which as out of Fountains, whereof the Nymphs were called Goddesses, water and humours do flow, & besides in them is all the joy and delight of Venus" (Sig. $D5_v$–$D6_r$/42–43). Sharp thus invokes the literary as well as medical language of the ancients, its nymphs and fountains vividly on display in a rhetoric concomitantly empirical in its clinical tendencies.

Even as she sometimes relies on classical authority to fashion her own, however, Sharp is not reticent about distinguishing an epistemology both practical and speculative from the more abstracted understanding of her medical forebears. The advantage of the empirical knowledge the ancients lacked means that Sharp can confidently distinguish her more accurate comprehension of the female body, and thus assert that the human woman's "matrix," as she calls the womb, "is far different from the Matrix of beasts." This is an important distinction "which Galen knew not" because of cultural restrictions that sometimes necessitated the privileging of theory over practice. Given that "the Grecians in those daies," Sharp writes, "held it an abomination to dissect any man or woman though they were dead; all the knowledge of Anatomy they learned, was by dissecting Apes and such Creatures that were the most like to mankind, but the inside of men or women they saw not, and so were ignorant of the difference between them" (Sig. $F2_v$/68). Even as Sharp emphasizes the value of the practical knowledge gleaned in her age over that of the ancients, however, she defers to the authority of the learned tradition they represent. Regularly invoking the teachings and the names of Galen and Aristotle, Sharp devotes an entire chapter to "Cold, Moist, Hot, Dry, and of all the several Distempers of the Womb" (Sig. $X5_r$/313), arguing that the ideal of balanced humours is compromised by wombs favouring one of the four, and throughout proceeds from the assumption that women are by nature both colder and moister than men. That Sharp's text colludes with even as it appears to resist the authority of both the learned and empirical suggests a discourse that is in some ways no less conflicted than that of her male counterparts.

Like the rhetoric of the physicians, hers also illustrates the inevitable interconnection of the medical and religious. Citing the example of physicians who "are at a stand and are never like to agree about" the fetus's *in utero* posture so that there are "not two in twenty that can set their horses together," Sharp invokes "the Prophet David" who "ascribes this knowledge as more peculiar to God, Psalm 139" (Sig. $L5_r$/153). Confiming the inscrutability of Sharp's "secret Cabinet of nature," the Psalmist writes in address to the divine that

> thou hast covered me in my mothers womb: I will give thanks unto thee for I am fearfully and wonderfully made: marvellous are thy works, and that my soul knoweth right well; my bones are not hid from thee, though I be made secretly and fashioned beneath in the earth; thine eyes did see my substance, yet being unperfect, and in thy Book were all my members written, which day by day were fashioned, whenas yet there was none of them. (Sig. $L5_v$/154)

Appealing to the persuasive force of an "Imagination" that "is powerful in all living creatures" (I5$_{v}$/122), Sharp recognizes the force of the patient's inner life in a medical epistemology that, insofar as its beliefs also depend on that which is not literally visible, is inherently linked with that of religion.[19]

For Sharp, however, medical empiricism transcends the limits of devotional imagination in discovering that which David could not. Though Hippocrates as well as the Danish anatomist "Bartholinus the younger" proposed to know that which scripture grants to God alone, Sharp rejects their imaginative conjecturing and concurs instead with the "expert Spigelius" and his visual rendering of the child *in utero*.[20] She does so not, however, by deferring to his authority alone. Rather, his drawing is credible only through verification by experience, through which she can confirm it to be "the very same with that of a child that I had once the chance to see when I was performing my office of Midwifry" (Sig. L6$_{r}$/155). The authority of midwiferly experience may ultimately trump the *aporia* of David, the speculations of Hippocrates, and the reimaginings of Spigelius, but Sharp's rhetoric cannot utterly divorce itself from the religious and medical traditions those devotional and medical authorities represent. Even when invoked only for purposes of refutation or support, their work allows Sharp to display her own understanding of the terms and tropes of the deeply textual epistemology on which her professional self-fashioning simultaneously depends.

A poet like Bradstreet and a healer like Sharp, physician Jane Barker unites the rhetorical and medical in the 1688 anthology titled *Poetical Recreations* and made up of "Original Poems, Songs, Odes, &c" along "with several New Translations." Offering "in Two Parts" a selection of poems by Barker and a secondary collection of verses "by several Gentlemen of the Universities, and Others," the volume showcases the accomplishments of a woman who could not have attended university herself but

[19] Recognizing with Bunworth and others the force of visual persuasion, Sharp also describes the "Jacob's Ewes" that had "conceived spotted, and grisled" offspring in response to the "peeled rods being set before them when they were in conjunction," as well as the ancient "Æthiopian" taught by Galen "to get a white child" by simply "setting a picture before him for his wife to look on" (Sig. I5$_{v}$/122).

[20] In her edition of *The Midwives Book*, Elaine Hobby confirms "Bartholinus the younger" as Thomas Bartholin, a "Professor of Medicine at Copenhagen," where his "father Caspar (1585–1629) had been Professor of Anatomy." *Bartholinus Anatomy; Made from the Precepts of his Father* was in 1668 published in a translation by Nicholas Culpeper and Abdiah Cole (119 n. 2). Hobby also identifies Spigelius as Adriaan van den Spiegel, who lived in 1578–1625 and was "the last great Paduan anatomist" (119 n. 5).

was taught physic by her medical student brother. Among the volume's prefatory paratexts is an address from publisher Benjamin Crayle. Offered with the "hope they may give as equivalent satisfaction as any that have preceded them" and confident of the work's quality, "the ensuing Verses," Crayle affirms, "have pass'd the test of several that know how to judge of Poetry, and that was sufficient to prompt me to the adventure" (Sig. $A3_v$). Confirming the popular reception of like anthologies as well as favourable responses to the previously unpublished verses within, Crayle makes a canonizing gesture not only on behalf of the university men the *Recreations* includes but also – and especially – the showcased efforts of a single (and perhaps singular) woman.

Though commending Barker's literary worth, Crayle does not mention her familiarity with the profession she would come to choose over poetry.[21] Barker does, however, use her verse to fashion a medical-professional ethos, and the collection's penultimate poem, "A Farewell to POETRY, with a Long Digression on ANATOMY" (99–106), sees her turn away from the "bright influence" (line 6) of "kind *Poetry*" (line 1) and toward "wise *Aristotle* and *Hippocrates*" as well as "*Galen*, and the most Wise *Socrates*" (lines 7–8).[22] Barker is confident that the ancient fathers of medicine will assist the journey she undertakes to visit "they with whom I must Acquaintance make" (line 11), who "will, no doubt, receive me for the sake" of the "*Him*" she footnotes as "my Brother" and "from whom they did expect to see / New Lights to search *Nature*'s obscurity" (lines 12–14). Drawing on the authority her promising brother represents, she goes on to present a vivid metaphorical tour through the human body. Like Sharp's discourse of midwifery, Barker's medical verse casts on the obscurity of

[21] Marilyn L. Williamson infers from a manuscript held at Magdalen College that Barker "was revising her poems at the end of the century" (103), some of which appeared in her later fiction. Barker seems to have left off both medicine and the writing of poetry, however, and in later works "represents her persona as ambivalent about women's learning" (103–4). Barker's Jacobite loyalties led her to France, where she lived until 1715 and "became an ardent Roman Catholic" (103). Religion seems to have preoccupied her for a number of years, and she produced little new work until the 1713 publication of the first of three novels for which she has become better known. Jane Spencer, however, identifies a collection of later poems by Barker held in manuscript at the British Library (Add. Ms 21, 621), titled "A Collection of Poems Refering to the times" and in which her speaker, Fidelia, "discusses public affairs in the years 1685–1700." Some of those poems, Spencer notes, are also included in the collection held at Magdalen College as MS 343 (179 n. 3). Barker was no doubt aware that "publication as 'literature' rather than as 'natural philosophy'," as Lynette Hunter and Sarah Hutton argue, was for women "far more acceptable, and clearly limited female involvement in technical and scientific matters" (5), a limitation that no doubt extended to matters medical.

[22] The poem is followed only by "On the DEATH of my Brother," suggesting perhaps the greater importance of the sibling whose own studies gave her access to learned medicine.

nature a new light of her own, making the unseen visible in a medical discourse that is at once learned and new.

Beginning with the musculoskeletal "*Architecture*" and concluding with a view of William Harvey's circulatory system, Barker's tour draws also on the mid-century contributions of Danish anatomist "Bartholine," who was "the first of all this Crew" that to the poet did "Nature's Architecture shew" (lines 15–16). Barker, however, presents the knowledge of "new medicine" in the metaphorical mode associated with its earlier age. Speaking to the poet through his work, Bartholin

> tells me how th' Foundation first is laid
> Of Earth; how Pillars of strong Bones are made;
> How th' Walls consist of carneous parts within,
> The out-side pinguid, over-laid with Skin;
> The Fretwork, Muscles, Arteries, and Veins,
> With their Implexures, and how from the Brains
> The Nerves descend; and how they do dispence
> To ev'ry Member, Motive Pow'r and Sence.
> (lines 17–24)

Invoking the familiar metaphor of human body as house, Barker renders the medical accessible and memorable. Delineating bodily strength evident in the "Foundation" of "Earth," "Pillars of strong Bones," and "Fretwork" overlaid by "Walls," Barker extends the likeness to include the "Windows" of eyes curtained and "trbly Glaz'd" (lines 26–27) as well as the digestive system's "Kitchin," "Dining-Room," and "Drawing-room" (lines 50–52).[23]

[23] Perhaps alluding to the scripture Sharp directly cites, Barker may have also been familiar with Mary Sidney Herbert's striking and then well-known translation of Psalm 139. Differing significantly from other translations, the countess of Pembroke's addresses the divine with an interuterine description more specifically illustrative of God's omniscience and the human body:

> Thou, how my back was beam-wise laid,
> And raft'ring of my ribs, dost know;
> Know'st every point
> Of bone and joint.
>
> (lines 43–46)

In contrast with Pembroke's *enargeaic* bringing-before-the-eyes, the KJV version offers the single, literal line, "I will praise thee; for I am fearfully and wonderfully made: marvellous are thy works; and that my soul knoweth right well" (line 14). It seems likely that Barker knew Pembroke's version, given that the seventeen extant manuscripts of the Sidney Psalms, as Wendy Wall explains, were popular enough to "become highly public texts, circulating wiely enough to be read by Donne, Lanyer, and Herbert, and surviving to be disseminated in the next centuries" (53) to be eventually published in 1823. That Barker knew other translations is further suggested by an interest in the genre evident in the *Recreations'* inclusion of her version of "Part of the XIX. Psalm" (56–57), one that likely encouraged her to read beyond those readily available in the KJV. (See Bennett, *Women Writing of Divinest Things* for a rhetorical reading of Pembroke's psalms.)

At the same time, however, Barker renders obscure the picture she paints, laying over with the grand what might otherwise be plain. Opting for the Latinate "carneous" over the synonymous "flesh" or "fleshy," "pinguid" over "fatty" or "oily," and the obsolete and rare "Implexures" over "An infolding" or "fold," the poet's elevated diction makes for a language more akin to that of the "elite doctors" whose "preference for esoteric Latin" (Furdell 81) was often met with suspicion by both patients and rival practitioners.[24] That Barker both speaks to and situates herself within an elite and exclusionary discourse is apparent also in an allusiveness recognizable only to those familiar with "carneous" and the especially rare "Implexure" that also appear in surgeon John Banister's 1578 anatomy *The Historie of Man*, a work likewise "sucked from the Sappe of the most Approved Anathomistes."[25] Given the difficulty or obscurity of her diction as well as her penchant for the figurative, it seems clear that Barker aims to assert her discursive place among the learned medicine's professors. At the same time, in both following the Paracelsian Banister's discursive lead and in its simultaneously plain and direct account of the literal bones, muscles, arteries, veins, brains, and nerves, Barker's style also favours a rhetoric of quantitative leanings. Thus representing tradition as well as change, Barker's mixed style seems equally intent on the literal specificities of a purportedly "new" medicine and the figurative conventions of a discourse more abstract and theoretical than hard empiricism may accommodate.

Thus rhetorically enacting Wear's continuity and union, Barker's bodily tour suggests a nuanced understanding of the profession in which she elsewhere explicitly asserts her place. In "On the *Apothecary*'s Filing my Bills amongst the *Doctors*" (31–34), Barker uses her own promotional flyer's inclusion among those of other physicians to fashion herself a healer as invested in practice as learning. Having taken what Patricia Crawford calls "the radical action of public advertisement" ("Advertisements" 69) in what we now recognize as the most persuasively intended of genres, the poet writes of her expectation to be counted among medicine's elite. Opening

[24] The *OED* points to the use of "carneous" in surgeon John Banister's 1578 *The Historie of Man*, from which also comes the single cited usage of "Implexures," and cites "pinguid" from clergyman and encyclopedist John Swan's 1635 *Speculum Mundi or A Glasse Representing the Face of the World.* All are Latin in origin.

[25] According to Andrew Griffin's *DNB* entry, the book also includes advice for treating pleurisy. Banister was a prolific writer who also produced *Compendius Chirurgery, Gathered and Translated Especially out of Wecker* (1585) and *An Antidotarie Chyrurgicall* (1589), and "his collected works were published in 1633." Banister belonged to a group of practitioners that historian Charles Webster allies with the Paracelsians, and his daughter "married the physician Stephen Bradwell," whose discussion of illness and fear is taken up here in Chapter 3.

with an appropriately modest gesture, she expresses the "Hope" that "I shan't be blam'd if I am proud, / That I'm admitted 'mongst this Learned Croud." Rather than taking up the anticipated *humilitas topos*, however, Barker resists also acknowledging that she should not speak above her reach, arguing instead, "To be proud of a Fortune so sublime, / Methinks is rather Duty, than a Crime" (lines 1–4). Recognizing the necessity of discursive belonging, even if only in advertising, she knows that "this 'tis, makes me a fam'd *Physician* grow" (line 13). Barker seems to know that the "Learned Croud" to which she refers not only endorses but also fashions the professional self. Pointing out that "*Saul* 'mongst *Prophets* turn'd a *Prophet* too" (line 14), she confirms the mutually constitutive relation of individual and discourse community – now rhetorically situated among the "Doctors," Barker implies, she may turn doctor, too.

Far from demonstrating the requisite feminine modesty, "On the Apothecary's Filing" makes the bold move of asserting that women are actually better equipped for healing, for "the sturdy Gout, which all Male power withstands," she writes, "is overcome by my soft Female hands." Displaying also her knowledge of scripture, Barker champions her healing art over the accomplishments of some renowned biblical women as she avers

> Not Deb'ra, Judith, or Semiramis
> Could boast of Conquests half so great as this;
> More than they slew, I save in this Disease.
> (lines 13–19)

Though professional self-realization comes only with acceptance as one of the medical elite, Barker does not align herself solely with "male-constructed medical authority" (Keller 108). A dozen lines later, she writes her hope that professional exclusion will be redressed by the accomplishments of women whose "case to *States-men* this our Skill imparts" will be so persuasive that "they'll force all Women to learn Arts" (lines 27–28).

Such an education would, of course, include extensive training in rhetoric. Merely implied here, the primacy of language to the professionalizing endeavour Barker soon makes explicit. Even as she admits a preoccupation with artful language that may impede professional focus, for she has "digress'd too far, so must return, / And make the *Medick* Art" her "whole concern," it is through poetry that she has "gain'd this mighty place" among the doctors of the poem's title (lines 55–57). Hence "In all our Songs," she will "its *Attributes* reherse" and

> Write *Recipes* (as *Ovid* Law) in Verse;
> To measure we'll reduce *Febrisick* heat,

And make the *Pulses* in true measure beat:
Asthma and *Phthisick*[26] shall chant *lays* most sweet,
The *Gout* and *Rickets* too shall run on feet.
(lines 61–66)

Though Barker recognizes that the physicians' intensely rhetorical orientation may compromise the healing they profess, she also argues that it is not the knowledge of "Febrisick heat," pulses, asthma, gout, and rickets that will establish and sustain her professional authority.[27] It is not the apothecary's filing of her bill but her skill in poetry, the art of "Wonders" (line 67), that ensures her place among the learned as it subsumes the medical into the "true measure" of verse.

That the artful use of language is integral to the practice of medicine as it is to ensuring the practitioner's place among the "Learned Croud" Barker suggests even in poems whose topic is not medical. In the lyric "To Mr C. B. On His Incomparable Singing" (76–77), the poet lauds the subject's "melodious *Voice*" (line 2) that brings "*atoms* joyfully advance / In happy Consort" (lines 5–6) and once-dead birds to life "with a *Song*" (line 12). Exploring the possibility of a reciprocal mind and body effected by song, the poet postulates that "if th' *Mind* upon the *Body* works / By secret *Sympathies,*" then we are also to ask, "who knows what in thy *Musick* lurks, / To cure all *Maladies*" (lines 13–16). The poet goes on to describe an effect akin to Collins's poetic "practise so pleasing," confirming rather than alluding to the therapeutic potential of song and, by extension, the verse that describes it. "If *Fate* this *Physick* shou'd prefer" (line 18), Barker goes on, her subject's singing the medicine of "all London and Montpelier, / Physicians shall exceed" (lines 19–20). The poem concludes that if what it postulates be true, then

Hence forward then let *Poets* Sing
No more of *Orpheus*;
Since we have one, whose *Voice* may bring
Health to attend on us.
(lines 21–24)

Moving music and verse from extolling the literary tradition classical Orpheus represents to the purview and practice of medicine, Barker

[26] Sometimes called *phthisis*, the *OED* defines the ailment as indicated by "Coughing or wheezing" and including "any of various diseases characterized by this, esp. asthma or bronchitis."

[27] "Febrisick" appears to be an adjectival form of *febris*, defined by the *OED* as a fever and used by Hieronymus von Braunschweig in *The vertuose boke of distyllacyon of the waters* (trans. Laurence Andrewe) in the first edition of 1527.

confirms the power of artful language to exceed in healing force even the knowledge that comes from the most revered seats of learned medicine.

Barker underscores the importance of language to healing practice in the poem "On my Mother and my Lady W–, who both lay sick at the same time under the Hands of Dr. *Paman*" (42–43). Further asserting her professional authority in passing judgment on the physician whose efforts evidently brought about the two women's recovery, the poem begins by likening the afflicted patients to "two sweet *Youths* strip'd naked on the *Strand*" (line 1) ready to embrace the "*frigid* Body" (line 3) of the "*Gulph*" (line 11) to the two women's "*Pious Souls*" (line 7) likewise prepared "to lanch into a bless'd Eternity" (line 10). Instead of "putting off the Robes of worldly care" (line 8) as they fully expect, however, the poet's mother and her friend are by their own "*Guardian Angel's* care" (line 5) saved "from the danger they intend" (line 6). Hence the titular "happy Paman" is "mightily approv'd" and "both by thy Patients, and the Poor belov'd" (lines 14–15). Extolling the attending doctor as the exemplary professional, the poet's apostrophizing injunction to "let no Slander light upon the Fame / Of thy great *Art*, much less upon they *Name*" (lines 16–17) asserts Paman's superior place among physicians, one upheld in contrast to the medical interlopers who are in no way his equal. "Nor to bad *Druggs* let *Fate* thy Worth expose" (line 18), the poet goes on in a passage that underscores the linguistic facility of the genuine physician in comparison with the mere imposter: "For best *Receipts*," she insists, "are baffl'd oft by those" (line 19) who can turn even the finest medical knowledge to dross and whose inept actions reflect poorly on the profession whose authority and superior understanding Barker upholds. Lest the unskilled "crop thy *Fame*, or haste thy *Patients* doom" (line 21), the elite practitioner must "let no *Quack* intrude where thou do'st come" (line 20). Worsening the condition it purports to address, such "Base *Quackery*" (line 22) is "to *Sickness* the kind nurse" and "the *Patients* ruine, and *Physicians* curse" (line 23). Defined not by gender but a lack of professional credentials and an inability to put medical texts to appropriate and effective use, the quack's ruinous treatments are bested by the "good" physician sent by "their Guardian-God" and "Who by his Skill a longer time them lent" (lines 12–13). Demonstrating a facility with language that at least implies that she would not err in quacking misreading of even the "best *Receipts*," Barker positions herself in concert with the learned physician of Paman's ilk and in contrast to the medical other.

No baffler of texts, Barker concludes in "On the *Apothecary's* Filing," she possesses the requisite command of rhetoric demanded by the profession she is therefore able to extol. Indeed, "such Wonders" she and her muse "will doe,"

> That to our Art Mankind their case shall owe;
> Then praise and please our selves in doing so:
> For since the Learn'd exalt and own our Fame,
> It is no Arrogance to do the same,
> But due respects and complaisance to them.
> (lines 66–71)

Emulating the model of "the Learn'd" in claiming the right and ability to exalt their fame, she pays her "due respects and complaisance" by taking up a discourse that sees self-praise not as arrogance but convention. Though Barker engages a rhetoric defined in large measure by professionals whose organizational ethos, Pelling observes, was "collegiate, not domestic" and "homosocial rather than familial" (*Medical Conflicts* 19), she is able to draw on her poetic and rhetorical prowess to fashion herself a participant in a discourse that may have been homosocial and collegiate, but could not utterly occlude an eloquent and learned woman. Though she could never be fully acknowledged a member of the College that defined the physician against all other practitioners, she is no "*Dunce* set up for Rhiming Quack" (line 30) of the sort she derides in "To my Friends against POETRY" (95–96). Not one to "wrack a *Metaphor* to death" (line 16), but familiar with both the Orinda (line 5) and Cowley (line 7) the poem to her friends invokes, Barker inscribes her place in the discourse of those who profess poetry and, by so doing, asserts her discursive belonging to the profession whose authority depends on the eloquence she also commands.

Though Barker may know as well as anyone that she may never achieve the true status of the learned professional, she nevertheless resists social and cultural expectations even when she appears to meet them. "A Farewell to POETRY" may end in the first of its concluding numbered stanzas by pointing to the divinity inherent in every "Art," including "Love, Musick, Physick, Poetry" (104, line 7), a change in focus reinforced by an altered line length and metre suggesting formally as well as substantively that there are higher concerns for both physician and poet.[28] Underscoring the

[28] Barker takes up religious doctrine earlier in the poem as well, where she refers to the role of sight in the Fall. "For 'twas the Eye that first discern'd the food," she points out,

> As pleasing to it self, then thought it good
> To eat, as b'ing inform'd it wou'd refine
> The half-wise Soul, and make it all Divine.
> But ah, how dearly Wisdom's bought with Sin,
> Which shuts out Grace, lets Death and Darkness in!
> (Sig. $H3_v$/100, lines 29–34)

primacy of immutable soul over changeful sense, the poem's doctrinal reiterations may get the last word but remain subordinate to the poet's interest in learned medicine. As much for Barker as "Eliza," it is through the body that the poet gains access to the spirit. "But now, my Dear," the stanza begins, "thou know'st more than Art can," and therefore also

> Thou know'st the substance of the Soul of Man;
> Nay and its Maker too, whose Pow'rfull breath
> Gave Immortality to sordid Earth.
> (104, lines 1–4)

The late seventeenth century was yet an age in which religion remained the most acceptable topic for women writers, and her poem of praise for Dr Paman ends with the wish that

> all the Blessings light on thee that can
> Attend a Doctor, or a Christian Man.
> Since by thy care thou hast restor'd to us,
> Two in whom Virtue's most conspicuous:
> Better, I'm sure, no Age can ever shew,
> Whose Lives are *Precepts*, and *Examples* too.
> (lines 25–31)

The "Christian Man" and the "Doctor" are as one, and for Barker the true physician embodies the precepts of religious doctrine made visible. "Thoughts to the Soul, if they be good," she writes in "To the Importunate ADDRESS of POETRY" (97–98), "are both its physick and its food" (lines 27–28). For Barker as much as her male counterparts, mind, body, and spirit are to some degree inseparable, and each commands the capacity to heal the others.

Denying the rhetorical capacity of women like Bradstreet, Sharp, and Barker, physicians like Bunworth also safeguard information that might orient the "ignorant" women readers they profess to "inform." Noting that he is "so farr from making collections out of Authours" while claiming to do so "on purpose for brevities sake," Bunworth's thoughtful concision also entails omitting "all those things in my own practise which I know to be familiar unto most Physitians," offering instead only that which has "not been hitherto published" ("To the Reader" Sig. $A4_r$). Willing to impart something of his own experience but not the texts or procedures that

The reference seems rather strategic, however, serving perhaps as the means to refute the notion that "Women know little, and they practise less; / But Pride and Sloth" their "*Counter-parts*" nevertheless "glory to profess" (Sig. $H4_r$, 101, line 37–40). Tellingly, religion and devotion are then abandoned until the formal and substantive shift into the poem's last three numbered stanzas.

define his profession's singular epistemology, Bunworth addresses an audience that may include women, but his audience implied is limited to those who already share his understanding. Justifying his refusal to lay open the deeper knowledge and broader application of learned medicine by claiming that women are as incapable of comprehending the discourse he withholds as the practical knowledge he presents, Bunworth is as invested in protecting learned medicine as he is in doing "reall service to the female sex" ("To the Reader" n. pag.). As "flattering" to the physician as it is "humiliating" (Fish 2–3) to the female reader, *The Doctresse* proves an artifact as self-consuming as Primrose's *Popular Errors.*

Women practitioners may have been excluded from formal medical training and derided by their male rivals, but the rhetoric as well as the reality of seventeenth-century medicine may not have been as exclusive as the physicians would have us believe.[29] As the work of Bradstreet, Sharp, and Barker suggests, women who wrote about medical topics may have been just as likely to position themselves in league with the self-styled medical elite as they were to challenge male counterparts and competitors, whether explicitly or by emphasizing the advantages of their gender.[30] More often concerned with professional status than gender politics, women who wrote from the healer's perspective also indulged in an authorial and professional self-fashioning that aligned them not so much with other women as with the physicians.[31] Taken together, the work of Bradstreet, Sharp, and Barker

[29] According to Weber, "Systematic harassment of female practitioners in England is not borne out by available statistics" (370), and there was not as much distinction between them and other practitioners as the physicians wanted to believe: Weber goes on to explain that "university learning created the physicians' monopoly and justified their high fees; but in reality, as Harold Cook observes, classical learning was the only distinguishing advantage of the university-trained physician, and the sole claim to his medical superiority" (375).

[30] Certainly, women who wrote on the topic often invoke a medicalized version of the humilitas *topos*, deferring habitually to the superiority of university-trained male physicians, but those same women sometimes also construe themselves as full participants in the discourse of medical professionalism. A necessary pathos, in other words, works in tandem with the speakers' ethos, claiming as it does the linguistic mystique crucial to a professional self-fashioning that depends, like that of the physicians, on upholding the difference between them and other kinds of medical practitioners.

[31] Hence the example of the seventeenth-century rhetoric of medicine reminds us of the limitations inherent in reading their work foremost as the product of women, a view restrictive in a context where even seemingly female-centred modes of practice may, as Weber proposes, represent a tradition more lay than gendered. Our tendency to assume otherwise may have led us to exclude women from mainstream medical practice more than was actually the case. As Weber argues, there was an effort to "preserve a body of medical knowledge specifically directed toward women and their needs" as an alternative to "university and classically-based male medical knowledge" (359). Hence, he suggests, almanacs like Sarah Jinner's and Mary Holden's did aim to challenge the medical status quo and are "similarly situated within a text-based classical tradition" (381). But such challenges were not exclusive to women, as "Culpeper's translations of Galen and the London *Pharmacoepia*" allowed both "men and women to access the medical knowledge of the universities" (376), and

further suggests that the boundaries of medical discourse and the profession it defined were more fluid than the physicians' exclusionary and often inflammatory rhetoric indicates. Even though "the trend of professionalization," Weber argues, would be "detrimental to women's interests from the late seventeenth to eighteenth centuries" (392), at least some women participated in that trend not only by inscribing their own place within an emerging profession, but also by fashioning the bounds of the discourse community into which they wrote their own belonging. Not only did some women who wrote from the healer's perspective participate in the rhetorical jostling that would ensure the learned physicians' place at the top of the medical hierarchy, practitioners like Sharp and Barker aimed also to distinguish their own brand of healing from that of others. Ironically, however, the rhetorical fashioning of self and other in which women also engaged helped move the learned physicians more clearly to the forefront of their profession as they increasingly took up the discourses and practices of their many rivals, including the midwifery that once belonged to women alone.

women healers followed van Helmont and Paracelsus as well as Galen. Thus, Weber infers, "gender does not seem to be a factor in determining a particular healer's praxis" (379). Women, Weber further suggests, may have become "folk healers" only retroactively, when nineteenth-century pharmacology began to isolate and use active agents instead of the herbs or plants from which they derived (379).

CHAPTER 6

"*A Bare* Physician *Stuft with Words*"
Women and Domestic Healing

Thomas Brugis's 1640 *The Marrow of Physick*, a "medicamentary" of remedies prepared "with little labour, small cost, and in short time," proclaims in its title page to be "usefull and necessary in any private house." Though books like his are "very difficult to be published in English," Brugis rejects the "eloquent and lofty stile" of "fancy delighting history" and writes the vernacular in "a plaine way to helpe the poorer sort" ("The Preface to the Reader" n. pag.). This "Practitoner in Physicke and Chyrugery" acknowledges that from the ancients "sprung the originall of Physick" (Sig. $B2_r/3$) but challenges its ongoing adherence to Greek and Latin while "a great number of people perish … when perhaps with a little instructions [sic], they might have cured themselves" ("The Preface to the Reader" n. pag.). "Rather of the Grecians minds," Brugis recognizes "that a good thing is the better, the more common it is" and therefore heeds the Ciceronian injunction not to regard "our owne particular profit, in keeping the secrets of Physick so close" ("The Preface to the Reader" n. pag.). Pointing out that there is "no disease can happen to our bodies, whereto the earth brings not forth a convenient medicine" by virtue of an all-encompassing "whole similitude" to the divine (Sig. $B3_r/3$), Brugis invokes Christian as well as classical authority to challenge the self-protective and self-promoting inclinations of his fellow physicians who, "knowing such things," would instead "be loath to publish them and make the secrets of their science common" ("The Preface to the Reader" n. pag.).

The sorts of remedies "usefull and necessary in any private house" were found also in the recipe books kept by every literate household in early modern England, some of which were published in best-selling offerings ranging from Gervase Markham's 1615 *The English Housewife* to the late-century publications of prolific Hannah Woolley, which included the *Queen-Like Closet* of 1670 and culminated in *The Accomplish'd Ladies Delight* of 1675.[1] Though most recipe collections remained unpublished,

[1] Laura Lunger Knoppers notes that "one of the most popular printed recipe collections in seventeenth-century England" was *The Queens Closet Opened: Incomparable Secrets in Physick, Chirurgery,*

that they were a staple of early modern households is attested to by numerous extant manuscripts offering instructions for cooking, cosmetics, and housekeeping as well as healing remedies often passed down from one generation to another.[2] A valuable household resource, the recipe books served as a repository for knowledge devised and recorded primarily by the women who kept them; hence "the early modern housewife," Jayne Archer notes, "was an important producer and consumer of chymical literature, knowledge, and practices" ("Women and Chymistry" 192). Many collections also incorporated recipes credited to other domestic healers, who were often higher-ranking aristocrats, as well as remedies attributed to one physician or another. Drawing on authority granted by class or profession, recipe compilers can thus be seen at least by association to fashion their own, while some, like the Elizabeth Bertie who appends "Doctor" on a title page that also includes the name "E. Doctor," are more explicit.[3] Most recipe books do not always impart so clear a sense of how domestic healers regarded their work within the larger medical context,[4] but they do bear witness to the self- and genre-fashioning "fluidity and flexibility" (59) Catherine Field

Preserving, Candying, and Cookery (1655), a compilation attributed to the exiled Henrietta Maria, who had nothing to do with its publication. The most substantial of the printed versions was, however, Hannah Woolley's later "ambitious recipe book" (Furdell 97), *The Accomplish'd Ladies Delight in Preserving, Physick, Beautifying and Cookery* published in 1675. The year was, Margaret Ezell explains in her discussion of authorial fashioning and the culinary, an intriguing one for recipe books that saw the reprinting of Markhams's 1615 contribution as well as no fewer than three works attributed to Woolley, including a supplement to her earlier *Queen-Like Closet* (1670). Though Ezell points to the difficulties of certain attribution in any case, the recipe book genre may have become more intent on authorial self-fashioning; as Ezell explains, those books "produced in 1675 in general proudly draw attention to the labour involved in assembling the recipes, the experience behind them … and the culinary inspirations of the author" ("Cooking the Books" 167), but this shift may have a great deal to do with an emerging culture of celebrity authorship enabled also by "printer, publisher and stationer" ("Cooking the Books" 175) and little to do with healing authority.

2 In the introduction to their edited essay collection, *Reading and Writing Recipe Books, 1550–1800*, Michelle DiMeo and Sara Pennell note that "recipe books or collections in print and manuscript" can be counted as one of the period's "most popular non-fiction print genres." Hence they are also "the most common forms of manuscript compilation to survive" (3). Some better-known examples include Mary Doggett's *Her Book of Receipts* (1682) and *Lady Sedley's Receipt Book* (1686). Now digitized by the Wellcome Library and freely available online, a number of manuscript versions have also attracted recent scholarly attention.

3 The MS is held in the Bodleian Library, catalogued as Eng. Misc. d. 435.

4 Most do, however, offer subtle information about how women writing in the genre "fostered a correspondingly fluid self constructed as positive, authoritative, and capable of healing (and being healed) through the writing, practice, proveing, and exchange of medicinal and culinary receipts," as Field suggests (59). Woman-authored collections not only, Field also notes, "repeatedly emphasize individual practice and experience of receipts" (56), but record receipts credited to one physician or another, perhaps in part to establish the credibility of the information they record as they inscribe their own place among the "doctors" with receipts of their own.

traces in her study of what Monica Green styles "an entirely new kind of women's medical authority" (290).

Proving Brugis's rule that "a good thing is the better, the more common it is," women's healing knowledge did win some recognition with publications that both responded to and fuelled medicine's popularization.[5] As much as popularizing physicians like Brugis, the authors and publishers who disseminated such practical knowledge entered into authorial as well as medical competition with the Galenic stalwarts who, Mary Fissell explains, persisted in seeing "themselves as medicine's elite" despite practising in a late seventeenth-century London "saturated" with vernacular medical texts and remedy books ("Marketplace" 126).[6] Challenged by expectations of accessibility as well as the healing success of their competitors, the ancient authority on which the physicians predicated their own was further threatened by the remedy books' popularity. Though the books' content was often directly or indirectly derived from the work of domestic healers, their recipes necessarily part of "the mental as well as the physical spaces of women" Archer describes ("Quintessence" 115), the

[5] Though most recipe collections remained in their originating households, scholars have done much to illuminate the practical as well as textual influence of early modern women's manuscripts. See especially Rebecca Laroche's *Medical Authority and Englishwomen's Herbal Texts, 1550–1650* (Farnham, UK: Ashgate, 2009) as well as Michelle DiMeo and Sara Pennell's *Reading and Writing Recipe Books, 1550–1800* (Manchester: Manchester University Press, 2013). Useful articles on the topic include Robert Appelbaum, "Rhetoric and Epistemology in Early Printed Recipe Collections" (*Journal of Early Modern Cultural Studies* 3.2 [2003]: 1–35); Penny Bayer, "Lady Margaret Clifford's Alchemical Receipt Book and the John Dee Circle" (*AMBIX* 52.3 [2005]: 271–84); Elaine Leon and Sara Pennell, "Recipe Collections and the Currency of Medical Knowledge in the Early Modern 'Medical Marketplace'" (*Medicine and the Market in England and Its Colonies*, Ed. Mark S. R. Jenner and Patrick Wallis [Basingstoke, UK: Palgrave Macmillan, 2007]: 133–54); Margaret J. M. Ezell, "Domestic Papers: Manuscript Culture and Early Modern Women's Life Writing" (*Genre and Womens' Life Writing in Early Modern England*, Ed. Michelle M. Dowd and Julie A. Eckerle [Farnham, UK: Ashgate, 2007]: 33–48); Catherine Field, "'Many Hands Hands': Writing the Self in Early Modern Women's Recipe Books" (*Genre and Womens' Life Writing in Early Modern England*, Ed. Michelle M. Dowd and Julie A. Eckerle [Farnham, UK: Ashgate, 2007]: 49–64).

[6] Given that "virtually all healers and sufferers," as Beier notes, "subscribed to a humoral view of disease and therapy" (31), this is not to say that women who wrote and recorded medical receipts did not understand or follow the premises of Galenic medicine. Grace Mildmay, for instance, offers a collection of receipts but presents the "goal of medical care" from a distinctly Galenic perspective, advising caution in acknowledging it a "dangerous thing to wear and distract the humours in the body by extreme purges or extreme cordials" (Pollock 110). Weber points to a similar merging of the domestic and Galenic in the medical receipts found also in the mid- and late-seventeenth-century almanacs of Sarah Jinner and Mary Holden, works that "did not offer an alternative female 'folk,' 'herbal,' or 'kitchen physick' medicine in contrast to university and classically-based male medical knowledge," though "their medical advice does represent a desire to develop, organize, and preserve a body of medical knowledge specifically directed toward women and their needs" (359). On the contrary, Weber notes, the almanacs' integration of discrete medical knowledge not only "helped to preserve classical knowledge" (359) but also confirms "the need for vernacular medical literature written by women" in a context that saw women "heavily involved in early modern health care" (401).

knowledge they shared was frequently appropriated – or at least mediated – by the men who ushered them to publication.

Competing with and complementing knowledge sometimes freely offered and sometimes made available against the learned physicians' will, popular publication worked to inflect a once-almost-exclusively theoretical epistemology with the practical and applied. In such a "context of theory change," Andrew Wear explains, the collections of healing remedies and receipts that appeared increasingly in print as the seventeenth century unfolded were also "given added force by the existence of alternative medical theories" as even physicians made "arguments for medicine to be open to all" ("Popularization" 30). Yet the staunch defenders of learned medicine well knew that "writing about medicine at all, let alone publishing recipes and remedies in the vernacular," as Elizabeth Lane Furdell puts it, "undermined the secretive traditions of the orthodox medical community" (83), and some remained intent on guarding their secrets closely as they discredited the "recipes and remedies" that threatened their epistemological authority. In a context in which remedy books were, like the recipe proper, "deeply embedded in early modern discourses of gender" as well as medical professionalism, their publication and production, Archer also notes, were necessarily and "intimately concerned with notions of appropriate female conduct, education and behavior" ("Quintessence" 128, 115).

It is on gendered appropriateness and how such notions are sometimes challenged but more often used to buttress the physicians' authority in the context of popular publication that this chapter focuses. Considering beliefs about appropriate female behaviour from the perspective of both genders, it begins by examining the attitudes of male physicians James Primrose, Edward Bolnest, and Marchamont Nedham toward domestic healing and remedy publication before going on to reveal some of the ways women's healing work is appropriated and mediated in collections as well known as Markham's *The English HouseWife* and Elizabeth Grey Kent's *A Choice Manual of Rare and Select Secrets in Physick and Cyrurgery* (1653) and as obscure as those published by physicians Edward Poeton and Owen Wood. Taken together, such examples suggest that women's healing knowledge served the rhetorical self-fashioning of the men who made it available, an end in part achieved by appealing to culturally accepted norms of feminine behaviour that women both resisted and endorsed. Suggesting something of the extent to which such notions were imbued in the early modern psyche, it turns out that the anonymous yet presumably female author of *The Whole Duty of a Woman*, a work dispensing advice practical and medical, does as much to uphold learned medicine's anti-feminism as female physician Mary Trye does to resist it. Such gendered thinking also allowed the male physican both subtly and overtly to lay claim to the knowledge of domestic healing, as evidenced in the work of physicians such as Thomas Cock, the title of whose *Kitchin-Physic* alone lays claim to an efficacy acknowledged with the proverb "Kitchen physic is the best physic" (Cook, *Medical Regime* 30), or of clergyman George Herbert, whose endorsement of herbal medicine likewise served the self-fashioning aims of a profession construed as exclusively male.

It is telling of the success of their rhetorical campaign that the physicians' protectionist, anti-domestic – and therefore anti-feminist – agenda is given voice also by those who were not their colleagues. Parliamentarian and poet Andrew Marvell, for instance, clearly registers his sympathy with the physicians in his prefatory tribute to Primrose's *Popular Errors*, where he allows women to minister only the innocuous "Cawdles, Almond milk, and broth" and prohibits them from tampering with the physicians' truly medicinal offerings. Limited to that which "The *Doctor* doth / Stint them," the poet reminds his readers that women "must not teach here" ("To his worthy friend Doctor WITTIE," lines 29–30). Had women not long devised and ministered a great deal more than "Cawdles, Almond milk, and broth" to the ailing, however, there would have been little need for either Witty's translation or Marvell's poem. Though the physicians insisted on ascribing to women healers the uneducated, unprofessional, and unincluded status Marvell reiterates, their proprietary injunctions speak to a reality quite different from the physician-privileging ideal the poem upholds.[7] Prohibiting women from healing practice meant denying that much early modern medicine was predicated on or borrowed from a domestic tradition largely developed and sustained by the "Housewives

[7] Women and domestic healers were sometimes granted grudging recognition by men. Even the woman-disdaining and staunchly Galenic Bunworth cannot wholly deny the merits of a hands-on approach very different from the theoretically informed treatments of learned medicine, including the example of physicians who managed to stay a seemingly incurable woman's "flux of bloud" with a napkin-wrapt toad "bound to her back" (Sig. $C2_r$), while Paracelsian practitioners adapted women's herbal and home-grown knowledge to their own healing practices, and Francis Bacon, as Keith Thomas notes, went so far as to admit that "empirics and old women" were "more happy many times in their cures than learned physicians." Like Bacon, other "scientists and intellectuals followed the example of Paracelsus and were prepared to learn from herbalists and wise women," and Hobbes also proclaimed his preference for "an experienced old woman" to an inexperienced but learned physician (Thomas, "Prologue"). Erstwhile medical student Robert Godfrey, who found fault in both the Galenic and chemical, addresses women's receipts more specifically than his famous contemporaries, advocating the "good" and "profitable" medicines derived from "the long experience of Mothers, Grand-Mothers, and Great-Grand-Mothers" through which "the Sick might be sooner reliev'd, than by such Recipe confused Medicines, as are commonly huddled into Books, and Printed through desire of Fame" (57).

and gentlewomen" who, Lucinda Beier notes, "were expected to be able to keep herb gardens, compound remedies and treat the illnesses and injuries of their families and neighbours" (29). Though learned medicine had long questioned women's healing practices even when borrowing from them, the physicians were further threatened by a popularizing movement that had gathered momentum to the effect that women readers, Elaine Leong explains, "fully utilized the offerings coming off the printing presses to extend, confirm and challenge their own medical knowledge" ("Reading Medicine" 577)[8] and responded with greater determination to claim the knowledge of domestic medicine as its female practitioners gained more ready access to what was once jealously guarded.

That the physicians' monopolistic desires required them also to take command of medicine's remedies and receipts the "Epistolary Discourse" prefaced to Edward Bolnest's 1665 *Medicina Instaurata* makes clear. Authored by political pamphleteer and fellow chemical physician Marchamont Nedham, identified on the title page as the author of that year's *Medela Medicinæ* and introducing a work professing to address "the Insufficiency of the Vulgar way of Preparing Medicines," the epistle expresses the belief that "our Art must needs be at a stand, while old Notions and Medicines are in fashion, and while old Authors are set up as the only Standard."[9] Suggesting an inclusive aim and challenging the epistemology of a strictly Galenic practice, Nedham argues that it behooves the profession "to try Doctrines and Experiments both Philosophical and Medicinal," a bridging of epistemologies suited to the book's intent to offer medical knowledge, as Bolnest writes in its "Poscript" [sic], made accessible through a "very plain

[8] Family recipe books, Leong notes in her case study of the Fairfax collections, can also reveal "how informal science has functioned in parallel to the goings-on in the academy" ("Collecting Knowledge" 97).

[9] According to Joad Raymond's *DNB* entry, Nedham was hostile to Presbyterianism and unsympathetic to Charles I, whose private letters he reprinted "with antipathetic annotations" in *Mercurius Britanicus*. A journalist and editor, he produced other newsbooks as well as *A Short History of the English Rebellion* (1661). In his *Medela Medicinæ*, "he argued that Galenic principles of medicine were corrupt and useless, that modern diseases were different from ancient, and that liberty should be permitted in the practice of physic in order rationally to develop new chemical remedies." As well as introducing Bolnest's work, Nedham penned the preface to Franciscus de le Boë's *New Idea of the Practice of Physic* of 1675, a treatise that "responded dismissively to some attacks on his works allegedly commissioned by the College of Physicians" (Raymond, *DNB*). Clericuzio explains that, as "the diffusion of Helmontianism in England reached a peak" in the 1600s, Nedham worked with George Starkey and George Thompson and "launched a violent attack on Galenic medicine." "As part of this assault," Clericuzio goes on, "in 1665 Helmontians tried to create a 'College of Chemical Physicians,' as an alternative to the existing College of Physicians, which obtained wide support from eminent figures of Charles II's court" (305). Nedham, in other words, was a vocal proponent of a shifting medical epistemology.

and Methodical Teatise in English" to those "whose sullen Fate, slender and mean Education affords them only the benefit of what is published in their own Mother-tongue" (148–49). Echoing Edwards's like invocation of Matthew's parable (25.10–14), Bolnest claims that he will "most willingly, for the good of Mankind" and out of implied Christian duty therefore "deliver the Talent bestowed upon me by Almighty God" (20). Virtuous in its professed aim and inclusive in delivery and substance, the book nevertheless presents a corollary advantage of exclusion valuable when, as Nedham puts it, "there is no way to redeem our Profession out of the hands of old Women, and others, but by setting the whole frame of Physick upon a new foot of Operative and Experimental Philosophy." As it turns out, the profession needs rescue from "vulgar Medicines" and "the hands of old Women" partly "because the common Methods and Remedies are every where to be had in Print" ("To Doctor *Edward Bolnest*" n. pag.).

Thus the publication of remedy books presented a serious challenge even to alternative physicians like Bolnest and Nedham who, says Harold Cook, evinced "contempt for mere academic titles" and resisted the hegemony of the London College's Galenist epistemology (*Medical Regime* 153).[10] Yet it was in part the efforts of men that gave rise to an exigence of professional redemption from the "common Methods and Remedies" delivered "out of the hands of old Women." Doing much to open the floodgate that would inspire Nedham's complaint, Markham's well-known manual, which offered substance disseminated by a man but recorded by a woman, was one of the most popular collections of published receipts throughout the century.[11] Claiming in the subtitle of the 1631 edition to

[10] Though it may be true that the hyperbolic rhetoric seen in the grandiose claims of some collections, as Seth Stein LeJacq in particular has suggested, implies remedy authors in direct competition with the physicians, most offer little in the way of authorial commentary. "Such quasi-miraculous cures" claimed by some recipe authors, LeJacq explains, "indicate that we should approach the question of the credibility of these claims for readers with care." "Nonetheless," he goes on, "recipes clearly indicate a broad remit for this type of healing" and articulate "a belief in the ability of that healing to outdo the work of physicians and surgeons" (460).

[11] Though other male-compiled resources appeared in the first half of the century, Markham's may be the best known among texts emphasizing healing knowledge and explicitly addressing women. Others include Edmund Gardiner's *Phisicall and Approved Medicines* (1611), physician William Langham's *The Garden of Health* (1633), John Partridge's *The Widowes Treasure* (1639), with its "sundry precious and approved secrets in Physick and Chirurgery," Thomas Bonham's *The Chyrurgian's Closet* (1630), while later contributions include Richard Elke's *Approved Medicines of Little Cost* (1651), A.M.'s *A Rich Closet of Physical Secrets aka The Child-bearers Cabinet* (1652), published by a printer named Gartrude Dawson, M.B.'s *The Ladies Cabinet Enlarged and Opened* (1655), which includes a section on "Physick and Chirurgery," James Cooke's *Supplement to the Marrow of Chyrurgerie* (1655), the anonymously translated *Compleat Doctoress* (1656), J. Deacon's manual to

contain "the inward and outward Vertues which ought to be in a complete Woman," *The English Housewife* invokes the rhetoric of religious obligation in delineating a woman who, "from the genrall example of her vertues, and the most approved skill of her knowledges," can show how "her family may both learne to serve God and sustaine man in that godly and profitable sort which is required of every true Christian" (Sig. $B1_v/2$) and through regular prayer also work to "procure Gods favour the more plentifully on all the household" (Sig. $B2_r/3$). Religious obligation is not, however, a pre-occupation but an entry point to the book's larger concern, the virtuous housewife's accomplishments that, as well as the "skill in Physicke, Surgery, Cookery" identified on the title page, include a long list of "all other things belonging to an Houshold" whose secondary status indicates the primacy of domestic physic and surgery as well as the cookery necessary to ensure health.

Promoting practical learning in a work that is also a repository for domestic knowledge, *The English Housewife* depends in large measure on the appeal of its logos. For that content, Markham does not claim sole credit, but reveals in his dedication to the dowager countess of Exeter that his is not "the full invention and scope of this whole work," and quickly points to its feminine (and aristocratic) provenance. Much of what the book offers, the nominal author points out, originated in a manuscript that belonged to the "Honourable Countesse," who was "one of the greatest Glories of our Kingdome." But Markham cannot and does not give the countess sole credit, and quickly reattributes the contributions of that "greatest" of "Glories" to masculine authority. The countess may have penned the manuscript, but the information found within, he goes on to explain, consists of the "opinions of the greatest Physicions which then lived" (Sig. $A3_v$). Hence the authority of the book's logos comes through a fashioned-by-proxy ethos that has nothing to do with the countess and her glories. Reclaiming the book's medicinal content under the purview of an exclusively male profession, Markham is even more specific in going on to credit the "two excellent and famous Phisitions" identified in the margin as Drs. Burket and Bomelius. Moving from the general to the particular, he proceeds deductively to discredit with the specific and concrete even the liminal authorship of the housewife countess, who now seems merely to have received the manuscript as it was "given to a great worthy Countesse of this Land." Though women in Markham's view are not

cure the flux, *The Charitable Physician* (1657), and, of course, various editions and translations of Paracelsus's *The Secrets of Physick and Philosophy.*

completely unsuited to the practice of healing, at least to the extent that they may "receive some ordinary rules and medicines which may availe for the benefit of Family" and thus present "no derogation at all to that worthy Art," they will never be in parity with men.[12] "Indeed," Markham earlier admits, "we must confesse that the depth and secrets of this most excellent Art of Physicke is farre beyond the capacity of the most skilfull woman" and therefore can be found "lodging onely in the brest of learned Professors" (Sig. B3$_r$/5).

Markham's elaborate maneuvering is not entirely effective, however. That he fails to persuade even himself that the countess played no authorial role seems evident in his need also to cast doubt on the book's content. In a self-defeating move that gives the lie to his earlier claims of male authorship, he does so by claiming the grounds of a failed logos. Insisting that the text does not offer the kind of information worthy of a true medical professional, he attributes an unreliable ethos to the woman whose own voice is suppressed and whose hand in the text he simultaneously denies, "as though," he says, "I would have her to assume the name of a Practitioner" (5). Markham's contradictory and self-defeating attempts to accommodate both the countess's social status and the anti-feminist tenets of medical orthodoxy make for a complicated and convoluted argument. Implying two incompatible scenarios, his explanation is difficult to follow. First, he suggests that the countess played a role in the manuscript's composition, which seems acceptable but nevertheless demands a de-professionalizing disclaimer, and, second, he argues that the mere act of her receiving and possessing the manuscript is enough in the way of feminine mediation to put its contents utterly out of the realm of reliable discourse. Regardless of which is the accurate answer – that the countess is acceptable as a mediated author or that her very touch taints the manuscript's credibility – Markham's specious ambivalence has everything to do with the need to articulate some widespread assumptions of feminine limitations that may have more to do with the very real threat of women's medical competence than any truly entrenched belief.[13]

[12] Edwards is less diplomatic in his *A Cure for All Fevers*, where he complains about "a huge swarme of petticoat Physicians and Chyurgians" who misapply treatments they have ineptly borrowed from the "learned and expert Physitian" on whom they eavesdrop: such "tatling" and "audacious gossips," he insists, should know that it takes "long time and great charges" to achieve the "deepe knowledge" of a physician (Sig. A2v).

[13] There are medical writers, like physician–surgeon Edwards, who sometimes acknowledge the merits of household healing practices. His critique of medical charlatans makes clear that alternative practices can even offer good, and he does not aim to "taxe nor ranke among this rabble of Idlers, those charitable and well-disposed people, which in the absence of the learned or expert Physitian or Chirurgion, do give some comfortable things." He also recognizes merits in medical knowledge

First published posthumously in 1653, *A Choice Manual of Rare and Select Secrets in Physick and Cyrurgery* offers a collection of the "late deceased" Elizabeth Grey's receipts that were evidently by a man "Collected." Appealing to the aristocratic provenence of its substance, the "W.J." who is likely William Jarvis presents in his dedication to Letitia Popham "this small Manuall; which was once esteemed as a rich Cabinet of knowledge, by a person truly Honorable."[14] The manual features the medicinal receipts "practiced" by the countess of Kent "widely noted," A. S. Weber observes, "for her skill as a physician and apothecary" that appear along with the "most Exquisite waies of Preserving, Conserving, Candying, &c." in its first edition. The 1655 second editon, however, to the original adds "several Experiments of the Virtues of Gascon pouder, and *Lapis contra Yarvum*" devised and included, the title page tells us, "by a Professor of Physick" (Sig. $A2_v$). Taking opportunity to disseminate his own efforts in work popular enough to warrant a second edition in only two years, the physician presumably gains an authority conferred by the countess's aristocratic status; bolstering the credibility of the contributing physician as well as the original publisher, her implied endorsement mediates and validates the authority of both.

The volume proper is made up of dozens of the countess's receipts offered with detailed directions and ingredients but, apart from those variously thought to work "with the help of God" (Sig. $E1_r$/49; Sig. $F2_r$/75), "by the grace of God" (Sig. $K6_v$/180), or "with Gods blessing" (Sig. $L7_r$/203), they are presented with little in the way of extraneous information or commentary from their putative user. Rhetorically, the stylistically unadorned volume relies for its persuasive force on a logos akin to Brugis's plainness

practically gleaned by those charitable healers "whose vertues or helps they know by experience to do good in the like case, to comfort a friend or a neighbor." Yet Edwards also makes it known that such intervention is permissible only "till better help may be had," at which time such "well-disposed people" need give over "all other to the learned and expert in those worthy faculties, who know best how to deale with them rightly" (*Cure* Sig. $A3_v$).

14 John Considine's *DNB* entry suggests William Jervis (also called Jarvis) as publisher, noting that the book "makes it clear in his prefatory matter that the collection was made by him for Elizabeth's use." Lynette Hunter includes Grey's manual among those that represent "one of the startling aspects of publishing in the 1650s" she identifies as "the sudden appearance of a group of books of scientific, pharmaceutical and medicinal texts by women," among which are included "Queen Henrietta Maria's *The Queen's Closet Opened* (1655) and Alethea Talbot's *Natura Exenterata* (1655)" (89). Hunter concludes that the latter's work "is highly significant because it documents the movement from a herbal-based Galenic medicine to a balance of herbal and chemical," thus anticipating "the new experimental science" while remaining as "rooted in the health care of her community" (104) as Grey's and Henrietta Maria's. Given the popularity of medical texts and treatises throughout the seventeenth century, however, I would suggest that their very small number may be the most startling aspect of the books' appearance.

that, in also avoiding "an eloquent and lofty stile," is likewise trusted to speak for itself. Both editions of the countess's receipts are, however, prefaced with the publisher's address "To the Reader," which proposes that "if thereby thou suck abundance of Profit, I shall be superlatively glad." Glad he might be for the book's potential "abundance of Profit," but Jarvis is nevertheless compelled to beg excuse for its substance. If "the effect not answering thy curious expectation," he elaborates, the reader will discover "upon a more serious reflex" and "know, that nothing is absolutely perfect," and goes on to explain that if there are "any, or perchance many unlooked for mistakes," they result from a "want of a due application." Pleading excuse for the book's less-than-perfect content, Jarvis places simultaneous blame for any resulting failures on an audience anticipated mostly to include the sex who had long taken charge of healing in the home. Even "the richest and most soveraign Antidote," he goes on to observe, "may be often misapplied," in which case, "the fault not being mine," the reader must "excuse & cease to censure." Ending in appeal to the pathos of a potentially misapplying audience, he asks for the "just, & but reasonable favour" of any sensible person that "thou shalt deservedly oblige me" (Sig. $B1_r$). As he deflects blame away from himself and toward the countess, whose own use recommends substance "collected, and practiced by the Right Honourable," Jarvis makes a gesture akin to Markham's in presenting a work associated with a woman whose actual hand in authorship is neither clearly established nor flatly denied, and he does so while placing the onus for any potential failings on the women who were most likely to use it.

Edward Poeton extols feminine accomplishment less ambivalently in the dedication to Francis, Countess of Exeter, that prefaces the 1630 *The Chyrurgians Closet*, an "antidotarie" offering receipts for various remedies "scatteredly set downe in sundry books and papers" by Thomas Bonham, his fellow "Licentiate in Physick and Chyrurgerty."[15] Commending the work unto the countess's "Christian and noble Tutelage," Poeton praises her capacity for healing. "For be it spoken without adulation," he *erotemically* asks, "where is there any woman living, that hath spent so much time in the study of this Art, and mad so gracious & painefull a progresse in the

[15] According to Cook's *DNB* entry, Bonham was a university-educated physician who (like Brugis) also practised surgery. Bonham is notable as well for "despite being a physician, Bonham took the side of the London surgeons in their disputes with the College of Physicians." In addition, Bonham authored a poem that "celebrated the work of one of the most prominent surgeons of London" and "in early 1605 he signed the unsuccessful parliamentary petition of the Barber–Surgeons' Company asking for the right to administer internal remedies."

practice therof, as your thrice noble selfe." The answer comes in the form of another rhetorical question:

> Do not the soules of the sick & sore, & the limbs of the lame, every where (where ere you reside) blesse you; proclaiming to the world, that *Exceters* noble Countesse abounds in mercy, charitie, piety, pitty, compassion, bountie, affabilitie, humilitie, hospitalitie, and all other commendable vertues.

Given the countess's numerous virtues, it is unsurprising to learn "that shee is constantly cheerefull in the diurnall and painefull performances of these fame-meriting actions" (Sig. A3$_v$), and Poeton's *epideictic* tribute constitutes high praise coming from a physician–surgeon whose colleagues are usually more intent on maligning women.

That the countess is likely Poeton's actual or hoped-for patron, however, may go a long way in accounting for the adulation he proclaims. Poeton also makes clear that she represents the exception and not the rule as he praises not traditional healing knowledge but the countess's "study of this Art" that is learned medicine. Poeton's dedicatee may have mastered the literary corpus on which the learned physicians predicate their authority, but he proves far more intent on enumerating and extolling the countess's "commendable vertues" and the praise of her beneficiaries than offering an account of the "fame-meriting actions" that define her healing practice. Fashioning a countess aligned with the abstract and theoretical, Poeton praises the knowledge she has studied but not the hands-on work of healing. Thus apotheosized to an ideal of abstract virtues upheld as unattainable by "any woman living" other than the countess, she functions as the *epideictic* vehicle that authorizes Poeton's own voice and lauds the physician's bookish epistemology over the practical exercise of virtue.

Fellow "Professour in *Physick* and *Chirurgery*" Owen Wood also appeals to female authority in his 1653 *An Epitome of Most Experienced, Excellent and Profitable Secrets appertaining to Physick and Chirurgery*. Proclaiming in the subtitle of its fourth edition to have been published "For the benefit of such discreet Ladies, Gentlewomen, and others which labour to do good in that Art, Mysterie, and Profession," the book has evidently been "approved" not only by "Doctors of Physick" Owen Wood, Alexander Read, and John Jonson, but "also by a skilfull Gentlewoman" identified as "J.S." (Sig. A4$_v$). Multiple editions and publication dates suggest that the work responded to the increasing demand Furdell identifies, a supposition supported in "To the Reader," where Wood, in noteworthy contrast to Brugis's 1640 complaint of a vernacular dearth, notes that "great plenty of such Books are published in the *English* tongue." But, as Wear reminds us, even practical writers of alternative camp "make the usual nod in the direction of the physicians" ("Popularization" 34). As it turns out, those English-tongued books serve an entertaining rather than medical purpose: "for we delight," Wood explains, "in uttering of *Pamphlets*, promising the revelation of secrets in *Physick*" in texts that "prove nothing else but triviall toys." Lamenting the many how-to books that had recently appeared, Woods objects to their popularity: "Many times we are reasonably ill stored with such stuff of late," he says, which has worked adversely to "emboldeneth no small number of bold *Knaves* and impudent *Queans* to meddle with the practise of *Physick*, to the utter ruine of no smal [sic] number of improvident persons, who commit themselves to the Skil and Cure of such unworthy persons" (Sig. $A3_r$–$A3_v$).[16] Wood aims not to encourage but correct a popularizing movement that affords "improvident" and "unworthy persons" the opportunity to profess healing.

Though his book provides information to a "publick view and censure" (Sig. $A4_r$) that will perceive its worth and thereby prevent the sort of "utter ruine" he describes, Wood makes it clear that publication also encourages what he means to decry, an effect contrary to his intent but one that corresponds with the aim of feminine inclusion expressed tentatively in the endorsement of the cryptic "J.S." and confidently in the book's stated appeal to "discreet Ladies" and "gentlewomen." Inclusion is not, however, the same as equality. "J.S." may appear among the names of physicians who approve Wood's work, but she remains anonymous and therefore separate and unequal, unwilling or undeserving of assuming a full-fledged identity whose revelation would lend no greater credibility to those of three men. Whether unknowing or deliberate, whether Wood's choice or the woman's, the anonymity of cryptic identification serves the gatekeeping proclivities of the medical elite; hence even a relatively accommodating text participates in the rhetorical exclusion upheld by the authors and publishers of other remedy books. Buttressing the physicians' established ethos by implying or asserting their superior expertise, such texts are mediated in ways that discredit both the physicians' rival practitioners and the women whose knowledge they occlude and sometimes appropriate.

16 The superiority of Wood's work to that of those "bold Knaves and impudent Queans" is further asserted in his invoking of the Stationer's approval of "this Treatise." Attesting to the popularity of his own text serves also as a gesture toward the emergence of a discourse community that more properly represents medicine as it should be practised: "therefore," he goes on, the Stationer will "not spare to publish Books of the like Subject as they come to his hands, if they shall bee thought worthy. For this is now the fourth Edition, and so well liked and accepted of, that three Impressions have come to sale in lesse then three years" (Sig. $A4_r$–$A4_v$).

Though possibly the product of a man, the anonymous late-century *Whole Duty of a Woman* claims in its title page to have been "written by a lady." Offering medical, cosmetic, and culinary recipes along with chapters of advice for living "from the Age of *Sixteen* to *Sixty*," the book is addressed to a female audience and presented as the largely unmediated work of the unnamed author. In its second edition of 1696, the manual opens with a preface "To Ladys, gentlewomen, and others, of all Degrees" penned by one who writes by virtue of "a Liberal, Education and many Opportunities to Improve what my Younger years were Seasoned with." Having "been no ways Neglectful to my self or others," the author goes on to claim both "Knowledge and Experience in such useful things" that "not only already have, but further will, prove Advantagious to both." Hoping to advance both knowledge and experience, she has left her work in the hope that it will "much Oblige Posterity" through "Seasonable Publication" only after she is "Resting in a Silent Grave" ("The Preface" n. pag.), presumably in the interests of preserving a now-silent feminine modesty through posthumous as well as anonymous publication.

Such an overarching attention to gender in a text "properly Adapted to our Sex" ("The Preface" n. pag.) extends also to the virtues of compassion and charity, and the author argues that "it is not alone sufficient that the Service of God is imprinted in our Minds, but it must be put into Practice" (Sig. B_v/2), urging the reader, "Let God be all in all with you" (Sig. $B2_r$/3). Drawing on the persuasion of Christian obligation throughout, the author advocates for the reader "a very commendable Industry, to qualify your selves to be helpful to the *poor*, in as many Instances as you can," which include "not only opening your *Purses*, but *Dispensatories*, to provid *Medicines* for such as by *Disease* or *Casualty* want that sort of Relief." The author would like to see more charitable healing, so "that our *Niser Dames* who Studey only *Cosmeticks* for themselves, would change the Scene" and cease focusing on the "*Reparing*, or rather *Disguising* their own *Complections*." Instead, the dutiful woman should "Study the Reparation of the *Decrepit Limbs* of poor Suppliants" (22), for "though it be less fashionable, it is a much better sight to see a *Lady* binding up a Sore, then Beautifying her Face; and she will cast a much sweeter favour in Gods Nostrils, with the Smell of *Unguents* and *Balsams*, then with the most exquisite *Odours* and *Perfumes*" (22–23).

Receipts for those "*Unguents* and *Balsams*" and sundry remedies begin to appear in the fifth chapter, following those offering copious and conventional advice to virgins, wives, and widows. The book's medical receipts are, however, introduced with no preamble or context. Though individual remedies do come with claims of being "excellent good against the Stone or Gravel" (Sig. $F1_v$/98), "a great Healer of the Stomach" (Sig. F3r/101), or "a great Strengthner of the Lungs" (Sig. $G2_v$/124), neither the book's nor the chapter's prefatory material makes any claims regarding their effectiveness. The chapter's epigraph does, however, defer authorship in styling what follows as "the Choicest and Approved Receipts, of the most Eminent Persons of this and former Ages" (96), thus predicating their authority on the eminence of those whose gender remains unknown. Even as it advocates "the Divine and moral Virtues" of women, then, the book works in suble ways to question the authority and efficacy of women who practise healing.

Despite insisting that women would do well to pay more attention to good works than good looks, the book's eleventh chapter focuses on the titularly promised "*Artificial Embellishments*" amplified in subtitular appositive as encompassing "*the Art of Beautifying the Hands, Face, or any other part of the Body*" (174). The author thus registers more ambivalence about the feminine quest for beauty as an undesirable distraction from the higher pursuit of tending to the ill than she earlier suggests. The author's renewed attention to beauty undercuts the incompatibility of cosmetic interests with serious endeavour she elsewhere implies, and does so to the extent that the book as a whole is ambivalent about whether beauty or charity is more worthy of attention. Going on to advise against overindulging in frivolous diversions, the author may suggest a virtuous aim when she maintains that gaming is lightly permissible, but "to do it often, to be call'd a Gamester, is utterly to be avoided," shunned only "next the things that are Criminal," but she does so while also stressing the importance of a woman's looks. The problem, it turns out, is not only possible association with "ill mix'd Company" and "a habit of Idelness," but that gaming might become so serious as to inflict damage on the feminine countenance. The author stresses the ill effects of gaming in her climactic and final point, warning that "if you should see your own Faces upon an ill Game, at a deep Stake, you would certainly desist from any thing that could put your Looks under such a disadvantage" (48). A "deep Stake" heightens the seriousness of what should be a mere game, and *gravitas* has discernible effect on one's "Looks." Though gaming may seem unrelated to healing, both can involve high stakes that might be equally incompatible with the feminine ideal the author upholds.

Ministering to the ill is, of course, at least hypothetically more grave an enterprise than tending to one's appearance. Nevetheless, the author at least implies undesirable effects accruing from endeavours that might include attending to the sufferer, whose needs are also supposed to supersede one's own interest in "exquisite *Odours* and *Perfumes*." *The Whole Duty of a Woman* may advocate that women command a healing knowledge they are morally obliged to share in practice and application, but the book also suggests that women would do well not to take their work too seriously. In this and in the deferral of medicinal authorship to other "Eminent Persons of this and former Ages," the text colludes with male authority at least to the extent that it does not claim even a small part of feminine authorship of receipts that include "Dr. *Butler's Ale*" (98) and "Dr. *Stephen's great Cordial Water*" (102) and strongly suggests that women inclined to take up healing do so only to their feminine disfavour.

Not all are so ambivalent, however, and the far-from-anonymous Mary Trye is forthright about championing the remedies included in her 1675 *Medicatrix, or the Woman-Physician.* Objecting to the "frequent Persecution" of the woman healer's "not only just and laudable designs, but even Charity, Christian Duty, and Goodness it self" (Sig. B_v/2), Trye claims her own command of "good Divinity, and reason" (Sig. B_v/2). In punning objection to the "*Verbalist*" who is "a bare *Physician* stuft with words," she insists that he is nothing without the herbalist, for "without good Medicines," the learned physician "is nor more to be regarded, then one of the Patients in *Bedlam*" (Sig. $H2_r$/99). Trye thus takes exception to the Galenists and their bookish epistemology as she aims to vindicate the work of her physician father Thomas O'Dowd, "a Chymical Physician, and Royal Licentiate," in response to "the Calumnies and abusive Reflections of *Henry Stubbe* a Physician at *Warwick*" volleyed in pamphlet war with the Royal Society.[17] Refuting the specious learning Stubbe defended against the new science, she reiterates that "a *Verbalist* is not fit to be decreed a *Physician* to the *Universe,*" insisting that "a Man may be a Schollar, and yet not Cure the Gout, nor many other great Diseases" (Sig. $I3_r$/117). Rhetorically questioning "how we shall be assured Mr. *Stubbe* is the only Man fit for this Lofty purpose," Trye argues that men of his

17 In one of the first scholarly discussions of Trye's previously little-known work, Stanton J. Linden points out that Trye's advocation of chemical therapy and rejection of the Galenic practice of phlebotomy offers a sustained " 'medicinal challenge' to Stubbe," and thus functions as "both a vindication and a challenge." The work, Linden goes on, may be best characterized as "a tribute to her physician father who died in the plague" and "a defence of chemical medicines and an aggressive attack on the man Trye sees as chiefly responsible for O'Dowd's loss of reputation" (342). For Trye, Stubbe is "the archetypal 'physician': academically and humanistically educated at university, formally trained in the traditional medical authorities which were read in Greek and Latin, licensed 'by bishops, universities and the Royal College of Physicians of London,' and occupying an élite economic and social position" (343).

persuasion offer only shadowy form and not the true substance of medicine, for "wince Words only will not do, for I see no Actions, without which, I am not oblig'd to believe what account *Stubbe*, and such – give on their own behalf" (Sig. $H2_r$/99). Championing experience over authority, Trye does not "wince" her own words in challenging an epistemology unproved by verifiable "Actions."

Among the lamentable "Verbalists," the book's title page points out, Stubbe is worthy of "nomination with *Cicero*." Trye makes clear that Stubbe's effectiveness in arguing against her father proves him a rhetor commensurate with the Roman orator, but she makes it equally clear that the "languages and Schollarhip" Stubbe "boasts of" make for a likeness not commensurate with Cicero's more commendable intentions. Rather, as Linden notes, Trye focuses on Stubbe's "ambitiousness, boasting, and self-praise" as well as the "taunting and ridicule of others" (344) characteristic of "an Age" Trye sees as "subject to Division and Subtlety" (Sig. $B3_r$/5). Hence, says Trye, "the Reader may see how small occasion, and mean matter" worked even to tempt "*Cicero* to swell in conceit," as he drew on his verbal skill to the dishonourable, self-serving end of persuading others "to believe such publick praises were due, and attributed to him, which in reality were not" (10). Fortunately for her own sex, "this Age being pretty kind to us," Trye is able to offer instead "a reasonable measure of sense" that constitutes "as much, and more, then he expects from a Woman," and does so hoping she will be excused for lacking "the vacancy of those Masculine Capacities he himself glories in" (Sig. $B3_r$/5). An "eloquent Opiniator" who must "depend very much on his Oratory," Stubbe needs to persuade even himself "to be absolutely and uncontrollably Doctrinal" (Sig. $B3_v$/6) in adhering to that to which Trye takes exception. Rejecting the blood-letting practice of phlebotomy, she promises that "skill and good Medicines will preserve and free the greatest Beauty, the finest Face, and most curious Skin form any mark, disfigure or pit of this *Beauty destroying Disease*" (106) in superlatives reminiscent of the emphasis on beauty that dominates *The Whole Duty of a Woman*. Like those she criticizes, Trye is not averse to indulging in excess while critiquing the physicians' abusive, self-serving rhetoric.

In light of her own "Medicinal Tender," however, Stubbe "must own" that "the medicines of *S. Helmont, O Dowde*" and others "are able to make better Physicians then *Galen, Kraft, M.* or *Stubbe*" and their Galenist confrères. Defending the chemical and practical over the theoretical and learned, Trye aims to validate the work of her father. To lend credence to her own contributions as well, the volume ends with "*An Advertisement of*

Dr. O. Dowdes *Medicines, and the Authors*" that draws on the professional ethos of the physician who taught her and a refutation of language's significance to the healing enterprise. Arguing that "since Letters and Words cure no Diseases, no not the Ague by spell," Trye professes to write not in service of her own profession but to the patient-oriented end "that the Sick may have some other benefit then [sic] Talk and Scribble." At the same time, professional self-promotion is not utterly out of mind. Like Barker before her, Trye "will advertise," but insists that she does so to uphold a healing ideal, "that as the great and only end of Physick is to preserve the Body in Health, and to restore it to Health when lost." Though Trye trusts in the persuasive power of her own rhetoric, language alone cannot do the job: "For what honour can he expect," she goes on, "that will write, say and avow those things he cannot, or will not make out and justifie." Words and book learning are nothing, and "what Physicians speak and write signivie little, if it cannot be attested by fact," the evidence and experience without which "their affirmations are denyed" (125–26).

Keeping her eye on the charitable aims of the right-minded healer, however, she turns from self-fashioning assertion to altruistic service. To the latter and higher end, she writes that "I thought my self oblig'd to give this notice" not only to those who hold the potential to fill her purse, but "to Poor as well as Rich and for publick good in general." Upholding the professional obligation to share curative knowledge, she shames the withholding physicians, offering instead "all the several Medicines of my Father, together with many others now in my Custody," which she promises "may at any time be had from me, by those, whose occasions require them" (Sig. $K1_r$). As "mistress of that Knowledge and Medicines," however, Trye claims to be uniquely equipped "to perform all this as far as the best of Medicines will reach." Like Brugis some fifty years earlier, Trye advocates on behalf of medicine's popularization as well as the charitable obligation for practitioners to serve all in need as she presents a sustained challenge to the tenets and practices of the elite physicians; like Brugis as well, Trye turns out to be a late-century exception that yet proved the rule.

The same year as Trye, Thomas Cock published his seemingly like-minded *Kitchin-Physick: Or, Advice to the Poor, by Way of Dialogue* including a physician, apothecary, and patient, respectively, named Philanthropos, Eugenius, and Lazarus. In the prefatory "Supplement to Kitchin-Physick" titled *Miscelanea Medica*, Cock proposes that too often "the Galenist and Chymist are represented, as two distinct, different and inconsistent things" and points to the falseness of such a dichotomy, for "'tis certain, they both serve but to make up one intire Artist" (4). Bringing together the theoretical orientation of learned medicine with chemical practice in the *Kitchin Physick* proper, Cock fully expects, "Now I am lanch'd," to see "nothing but storm and tempest," and points to the acquisitive ends of those who would claim that medicines are "not *good*" because they are also affordable. Anticipating economically motivated objections, he counters with a Christian platitude pointing to the implication that to believe as much is also to imply that "God had not ordain'd things *necessary* for the preservation of the poor, as well as rich" (Sig. $B3_r$/5). Yet dissenting practitioners "for want of better arguments" may "cavil at the subject matter, esteeming it below the state and *Grandeur* of a Physician," deeming the proffered receipts "more fit for some waiting Gentlewoman, Nurse, or Master of the Pantry" (Sig. $B4_r$/7).

Cock makes it clear that the debate between the university-educated and hands-on practitioners had not yet been laid to rest as he insists that the physicians' anticipated counter argument "savours so strong of calumny, design and arrogancy; that it stinks alive, and stands in need of nothing, but contempt and scorn" (Sig. $B4_r$/7). Worse, the poor suffer as a result, insists Cock, "because Colledge [sic] Physicians, and such as are approved, and have been Educated in the Universities, do not take more care of the poor; it being not in their power to pay both for *Advice* and *Physick*" (Sig. B_v/2). That the rhetoric of learned medicine was late in the century yet intent on upholding the physicians' bookish and therefore superior training Cock underscores as he invokes scripture in anticipation that some others "would fain say something, will 'tis likely tell you, the dress and stile is too plain and poor, too mean, faint and feble, to contend and meddle with *Goliah* among the Philistins" (Sig. $B3_v$/6). The credibility that accrues to eloquence some attach also to a knowledge of ancient languages; unlike such gatekeepers, however, Cock sees no point in requiring readers to learn Greek "only to understand the Title page of a Book" or to put them off with discourse that deliberately works to exclude, for he does "hate that sneaking trick with daring, doubtful, and difficult *words* to confound *sense*, hoping thereby to make them pass for *reason*" (Sig. $B3_v$/6). As much as Cock may style himself a champion of those he prays "God defend and keep from danger and delusion" (15), however, he is not free from some of his antecedents' familiar biases. Defending those who cannot access medical information for want of education or cannot attain proper care for lack of money, given that it is the unfortunate combination of both that sees "poor people run headlong to Mountebanks, silly Women, Mechanicks, Pseudo-Chymists, and their Graves" (Sig. $B4_v$/8), Cock persists in upholding the medical-professional divide insisted upon by the physicians. What may be most telling of Cock's work, however, is not his objection to the impracticality of a university education for the practice of medicine, but that a book titled *Kitchin Physick* includes "silly Women" among the quacks who send dupes to their graves.

Those who practise "kitchen physic" are sometimes subordinated also to the cleric who may, like Herbert in his *Country Parson*, acknowledge the value of domestic healing traditions but asserts the primacy of a profession exclusively male. Fashioning a parson poised not only to acquire with ease the physician's book learning, Herbert also claims under his purview an easily acquired and applied understanding of the production and application of medicine. Armed with the knowledge imparted by a mere "one herbal" (235), the ideally multitasking parson also takes up the role of the domestic healer. Herbert does profess that "instead of the qualities of the world" the parson asks of his wife "no other but to have the skill of healing a wound or helping the sick" (235) but, whether acting in place of or with the women whose gardens and recipes had long provided treatments for myriad ailments, such practical work cannot take precedence. Rather,

> now both the reading of him and the knowing of herbs may be done at such times as they may be an help and a recreation to more divine studies, Nature serving Grace both in comfort of diversion and the benefit of application when need requires; as also by way of illustration, even as our Saviour made plants and seeds to teach the people: for he was the true household, who bringeth out of his treasure things new and old, the old things of philosophy and the new of Grace, and maketh the one serve the other. (235)

Herbert therefore does not set his parson in opposition to the female healer with her "home-bred medicines" (236) or the apothecary, as the physicians so often do. Yet Herbert attaches even less difficulty to acquiring the knowledge of the herbalist than that of the physician, and both are subordinate to the role of the cleric. The healing occupation may even be as recreational as it is serious, with the results serving as "help" to but not replacement for "divine studies." In this view, bodily healing functions as a mere adjunct to concerns that are spiritual, and so is the work of the women implied.

Reading the advocated "knowing of herbs" as evincing Herbert's endorsement of collaborative or perhaps equal work in marriage, Cooley observes the passage's affirmation that "the parson's duties as a healer are to be delegated to, or shared with, his wife." Going on to note that "in the context of the gradual exclusion of women from medical practice in early modern Europe," Cooley concludes that Herbert's position on domestic healing "is worthy of comment" (68). Though Cooley does not specify how we might read the proffered recommendation in the context of the woman healer's "gradual exclusion" from practice, it is arguable that Herbert merely takes with one hand what he seems to give with the other. Herbert, in other words, may acknowledge the merits of women's healing knowledge, but simutaneously negates it in laying claim to their healing practice and, more importantly, subordinating it to the divine calling of the parson. As Cooley writes of "Herbert's rhetoric" earlier in his discussion of *The Country Parson*'s negotiation with the professions of medicine and law, it is at once and "alternately exclusive and inclusive, uncompromising and conciliatory, identifying and differentiating" (38). Such an alternating and sometimes concomitant duality applies as much to Herbert's treatment of women and the work on which the parson's interdisciplinary knowledge in part depends.

What Herbert's vacillating also suggests is that the hierarchy construed by licensed professionals who strove to place themselves firmly on top belies a practical reality that resists easy categorization and firmly defined allegiances. Visible also in male negotiations with and appropriation of medical knowledge gleaned from remedy books that included women's, "the narrative of exclusion and subjugation solidifies a tripartite division" among physicians, surgeons, and apothecaries that, as Rebecca Laroche shows in her study of sixteenth- and seventeenth-century herbals, "was not historically in place" (5).[18] As it worked to fashion distinctions among medical practitioners, the rhetoric of learned medicine sought to uphold the division of women from the male physicians who increasingly laid claim to aspects of medical practice antithetical to an epistemology that remained staunchly Galenic. Along with the continuity and union Wear identifies, then, there is also much evidence of change in the decades following the vitriol of John Cotta's 1612 attack on meddling women.

[18] In *Medical Authority and Englishwomen's Herbal Texts, 1550–1650*, Laroche aims to demonstrate "how both male-authored and female-authored writings represent women's herbal practice as constituting various relationships with medical authority, which itself was paradoxically both solidified and made fluid through publication" (9). As well as examining the various inscriptions made in women's herbals, Laroche considers how writers like Margaret Hoby, Grace Mildmay, Elizabth Isham, and Isabella Whitney attest to the usefulness of their own herbal reading in the context of her third chapter's titular "absent-present physician," thus representing "more and other than the general cultural phenomenon of women's medicine" (10). Though Laroche touches on topics rhetorical, as when she considers the "rhetorical moves" prefatory to the intently gendering sixteenth-century herbals of William Turner (29), her study focuses on the reception and the effects of the books' ownership rather than the discursive negotiation of professional definition and status.

Predicating his argument on an ethos fashioned by contrast, Cotta insisted that "because God and nature" had not endowed women with the requisite "learned reason and understanding" to aspire to the physician's knowledge, "their authority in learned knowledge cannot be authenticall" and women who deigned to practise healing could only be the worst of presumptuous practitioners. "In cases of life and death," therefore, "there ought to be no daring or attempts at all," and physicians are right to be wary of women's "dangerous whisperings about the sicke" (25). Ironically, those dangerous whisperings grew increasingly credible and public even as the physicians' claims to dominion became ever more firmly entrenched. As much as their rhetoric may have enabled a monopolizing quest that included taking charge of the once-exclusively-feminine art of midwifery, the seventeenth-century physicians could lay no firmer claim to the practice of healing any more than they held sole command of the verbal art so key to staking their self-fashioning claims. Whether finding a measure of agency in writing about or through illness, shaping their own professionalizing ethos as they engaged the discourse of learned medicine, or recording medical advice in their receipt books, seventeenth-century women knowingly and actively participated in debates and discourses that may have aimed to subordinate and exclude but also proved the physicians' end not easily won.

Conclusion

Though Beier may be right to argue that "there was no seventeenth-century medical profession" (255), there is little question that the physicians came to dominate the one that was emerging, and there is also "little doubt," as Horobin puts it, that latter-day physicians have succeeded "in establishing high status, protection from lay criticism and favourable terms on which to define and monopolise." That even today "medical work is what medical workers say it is" (90) attests to the success of the physicians' self-fashioning enterprise; that even today the "charismatic elements" Horobin also sees as integral to upholding the profession's prestige rely on the "morality" and "mystery" (95) that in large measure defined modern medicine's seventeenth-century antecedent attests to a profession yet dependent on ethical persuasion and protected knowledge. It may be that early modern medicine "was a profession of quite different characteristics" than the one Freidson argues "is less than a hundred years old" (5), but the discourse that upholds the latter-day physicians' insistent distinctiveness remains the product of anxieties not so different from those of their early modern counterparts. Equally aware that, as Horobin explains in parenthetical amplification, "the more we know, the more we realise how much more there is to know" (95), modern medicine may also share the early modern humanist's simultaneous pride and despair.

The seventeenth-century physicians' persuasive success in the face of uncertainty may come as no surprise given a medical education that included extensive training in rhetoric. But this is not to say their task was an easy one, and the physicians needed to contend not only with rival clerics and empirics, but also with the women who knowingly and capably participated in early modern medicine. Partly in response to such pressures and despite proclaimed allegiance to tradition, the profession staked by the early modern physicians was also developing "a new style of enquiry" that moved slowly away from a theoretical, bookish understanding and toward a more practical, and even empiricist, epistemology. Though Galenism's influence would endure far beyond the seventeenth century, by the mid-eighteenth, medical treatises "appear to have become less theoretically stringent and more reflective of actual practice through implementing a greater focus on patient care" and, Churchill also points out, less interested in emphasizing "practitioner expertise and authority" (232). That their profession would need to change to secure the physicians' preeminence, and that it needed to do so partly in response to the efforts of their rivals, seemed clear even when Cotta penned his 1612 diatribe. As Harley notes, "Whenever a new style of enquiry is developed, a rhetorical campaign is required to legitimate it and differentiate it from earlier styles," and there is no question that Cotta and other physicians worked very hard to legitimate and differentiate a discipline at the cusp of a paradigm shift as they fortified their professional enclave. Given that "disciplinary histories, new vocabulary, and new forms of discourse are the methods of pursuing such ends" (Harley, "Social Construction" 411) and, if new vocabulary is the hallmark of an emerging or changing discipline, then even Cotta's 1612 treatise anticipated what was to come. An "energetic snapper-up of new coinages," as R. W. McConchie observes, Cotta is credited with contributing several dozen additions to the *OED*, not all of which are the "latinate neologisms" we might expect from a university-trained physician.[1] That few of Cotta's contributions are exclusively medical terms, and include words not listed in the *OED* surely suggests an uneasy struggle to find a language equal to preserving the mystery so key to the physicians' self-fashioning, the "keeping the secrets of Physick so close" to which Brugis would object in 1640.

As much as it served learned medicine's self-fashioning, however, the obfuscations of mystery may have also impeded a profession whose autonomy, Freidson argues, rendered medicine "blind to its own shortcomings" even as it "facilitated the improvement of scientific knowledge about disease and its treatment" (371). Though Freidson writes about modern medicine, it may also be true that the early modern physicians' insistence on the autonomy afforded by archetypal exceptionalism likewise blinded them to shortcomings only acknowledged in the eventual – and slow – adoption of the empiricism they once disdained. No longer regarded as "a matter of the gradual accumulation of truth," writes Grant Gillett in summarizing the shift effected by Thomas Kuhn, science "is marked by revolutions"

[1] That in 1654 the professed "Doctor of Physick" John Bulloker *published An English Expositor: Teaching the Interpretation of the hardest words used in our Language* with "sundry Explications, Descriptions, and Discourses" further suggests the learned physicians' interest in language.

that see "old paradigms" sometimes "attacked, ravaged and discarded" and sometimes "abandoned through creeping disaffection as new paradigms are erected in their place" (287). There is no question that learned medicine was under attack in the seventeenth century, but the response might be more accurately described as the discursive manifestation of the physicians' "creeping disaffection" rather than the outright discarding of theory or praxis, given that little actually changed for "the individual sufferer" even in the century long regarded as "a watershed in the development of English medicine" (Beier 7) – it is well known that Galenism served as the cornerstone of medical theory and practice for at least another hundred years.[2] Fuelled by the "anxieties and distrust" of early modern medicine, says Porter, physicians of a long century that began in the seventeenth struggled to assert their authority as they competed in an ongoing agon of "Rival doctors" who yet "seemed ever at cuffs." As the eighteenth century unfolded to confirm that the physicians' "imagery of self-promotion," as Porter notes, remained "dependent on fashion," the requisite "revamping of images" (*Bodies Politic* 208–9) both verbal and visual suggests an ongoing self-fashioning set in motion by their antecedents and necessitated by practical shortcomings that were as obvious as they were troublesome.

Like any other, "medicine bases its claim to be a profession on several grounds," but its status requires that the claim be "honoured by the public on similar grounds" (Horobin 94). That the physicians understood that their profession would not have acquired its status without public assent is surely attested to by the frequency and vehemence of their professionalizing arguments, yet their concern for an audience whose approval they needed to win and not merely coerce may have emerged only as the profession became increasingly besieged. That Walter Cary in 1587 requested indulgence from a readership asked "not rashlie to condemne me" surely anticipates a need that only later became fully realized. Inviting readers discerning anything "thou mislike" to "write thy mind, and deliver it to the printer," Cary promises response to such criticisms, and claims to "be verie willing, by writing againe to satisfie thee; or otherwise thankfullie to accept thine advise, and confesse my fault." Cary does, however, recognize that his offering of "diverse good and perfect remedies" defies professional norms of discourse and practice as he admits that "both in the description

[2] Historians generally agree that modern medicine emerged only in the nineteenth century. David Wootton suggests the application of Lister's germ theory in 1865 as the moment when medical epistemology (if not medical therapy) began effectively to change: hence it wasn't until "the medical revolution of the nineteenth century," he notes, that "textbooks were no longer restatements of the teachings of Hippocrates and Galen" (Intro.)

(desiring to be more plaine) and cure thereof, I digresse somewhat from manie writers" (Sig. Aiij$_r$–Aiij$_v$). Though Cary offers only the cryptic "sundrie causes" for bidding his *Farewell to Physic*, it may be that a "master of Arts" and "student in physicke," who writes in a plain style and values the non-medical reader through at least six editions, held inclinations too populist to suit the ethos and mystery upheld by learned medicine well into the seventeenth century and beyond.

Works Cited

Abernethy, John. *A Christian and Heavenly Treatise: Containing Physicke for the Soule*. 3rd edn. London: Richard Badger, 1615. *Early English Books Online*. 25 July 2013.

Adams, Thomas. *Diseases of the Soule: A Discourse Divine, Morall, and Physicall*. London: George Purslowe, 1616. *Early English Books Online*. 16 October 2013.

Albury, W. R. "Broadening the Vision of the History of Medicine." *Health and History* 7.1 (2005): 2–16. JSTOR. 5 August 2010.

Allen, D. E. "Merret, Christopher (1614–1695)." *Oxford Dictionary of National Biography*. Oxford: Oxford UP, 2004; online edn, May 2006. 8 March 2013.

Anon. *The Compleat Doctoress: Or, A Choice Treatise of All Diseases Insident to Women*. London: Edward Farnham, 1656. *Early English Books Online*. 27 May 2008.

Philiatros, Or the Copie of an Epistle, wherein sundry fitting Considerations are Propounded to a young Student of Physicke. London: W. White, 1615. *Early English Books Online*. 27 May 2008.

The Whole Duty of a Woman: Or a Guide to the Female sex from the Age of Sixteen to Sixty, &c. 2nd edn. London: J. Gwillim, 1696. *Early English Books Online*. 31 May 2013.

Archer, Jayne Elisabeth. "The 'Quintessence of Wit': Poems and Recipes in Early Modern Women's Writing." In DiMeo and Pennell, 114–34.

"Women and Chymistry in Early Modern England: The Manuscript Receipt Book (c. 1616) of Sarah Wigges." *Gender and Scientific Discourse in Early Modern Culture*. Ed. Kathleen P. Long. Burlington VT: Ashgate, 2010. 191–216.

Aristotle. *On Rhetoric*. Trans. George A. Kennedy. New York and Oxford: Oxford University Press, 1991.

Astell, Mary. *Six Familiar Essays upon Marriage, Crosses in Love, Sckness, Death, Loyalty and Friendship*. London: Tho. Bennet, 1696. *Early English Books Online*. 18 August 2010.

Axtell, James L. "Education and Status in Stuart England: The London Physician." *History of Education Quarterly* 10.2 (1970): 141–159. *JSTOR*. 7 July 2010.

Banister, John. *The Historie of Man, Sucked from the Sappe of the most Approved Anathomistes*. London: John Daye, 1578. *Early English Books Online*. 21 October 2013.

Barker, Jane. *Poetical Recreations*. London: Benjamin Crayle, 1688. *Early English Books Online*. 27 March 2012.

Baumlin, James S. and Tita French Baumlin. "Psyche/Logos: Mapping the Terrains of Mind and Rhetoric." *College English* 51.3 (1989): 245–61. *JSTOR*. 28 January 2013.

Baxter, Richard. *Reliquiæ Baxterianæ: Or, Mr. Richard Baxters Narrative of the Most Memorable Passages of His Life and Times*. London: Matthew Sylvester, 1696. *Early English Books Online*. 16 June 2011.

Beier, Lucinda McCray. *Sufferers and Healers: The Experience of Illness in Seventeenth-Century England*. London and New York: Routledge & Kegan Paul, 1987.

Bennett, Lyn. "Negotiating the Public and the Private: Rhetoric and Women's Poetry in Interregnum England." *Rhetor* 4 (2011). 15 October 2012.

Women Writing of Divinest Things: Rhetoric and the Poetry of Pembroke, Wroth, and Lanyer. Medieval and Renaissance Studies Series. Pittsburgh: Duquesne University Press, 2004.

Berensmeyer, Ingo. "Rhetoric, Religion, and Politics in Sir Thomas Browne's *Religio Medici*." *SEL: Studies in English Literature 1500–1900*. 46.1 (2006): 113–32. *Project Muse*. 30 December 2010.

Berg, Christine and Philippa Berry. "'Spiritual Whoredom': An Essay on Female Prophets in the Seventeenth Century." *1642: Literature and Power in the Seventeenth Century*. Ed. Francis Barker et al. Essex: University of Sussex Press, 1981. 11–36.

Bertie, Elizabeth. *Elizabeth Bertie: Her Booke*. Oxford: Bodleian Library: MS Eng. Misc. d. 435.

Bewick, John. *An Antidote against Lay-Preaching*. London: Andrew Crook, 1642. *Early English Books Online*. 16 October 2013.

Bible. King James Vers.

Bicks, Caroline. "Stones like Women's Paps: Revising Gender in Jane Sharp's Midwives Book." *Journal for Early Modern Cultural Studies* 7.2 (2007): 1–27. *JSTOR*. 12 May 2013.

Birken, William. "The Dissenting Tradition in English Medicine of the Seventeenth and Eighteenth Centuries." *Medical History* 39:2 (1995): 197–218. *ProQuest*. 17 July 2009.

Blackstock, Carrie Galloway. "Anne Bradstreet and Performativity: Self-Cultivation, Self-Deployment. *Early American Literature* 32.3 (1997): 222–48.

Bloomquist, L. Gregory. "Subverted by Joy: Suffering and Joy in Paul's Letter to the Phillipians." *Interpretation* 61.3 (2007): 270–82.

Blount, Thomas. *The Academie of Eloquence*. London: T. N. for Humphrey Moseley, 1654. *Early English Books Online*. 21 August 2008.

Bolnest, Edward. *Medicina Instaurata, or; A Brief Account of the true Grounds and Principles of the Art of Physic*. London: John Starkey, 1665. *Early English Books Online*. 3 June 2008.

Bonham, Thomas. *The Chyrurbians Closet: Or, An Antidotarie Chyrurgicall*. London: George Miller, 1630. *Early English Books Online*. 3 June 2008.

Bono, James J. *The Word of God and the Languages of Man: Interpreting Nature in Early Modern Science and Medicine.*Madison: University of Wisconsin Press, 1995.

Boorde, Andrew. *The Breviarie of Health.* London: Thomas Este, 1598. *Early English Books Online.* 3 June 2008.

Boswell, James. *Life of Johnson.*1791. Oxford: Oxford University Press, 1980. 18 May 2013.

Brackett, Virginia. "The Countesse of Lincolne's Nurserie as Inspiration for Anne Bradstreet." *Notes and Queries* 42.240 (1995): 364–65.

Bradstreet, Anne. *The Tenth Muse.* London: Stephen Bowtell, 1650. *Women Writers Online.* 6 March 2012.

The Works of Anne Bradstreet. Ed. Jeannine Hensley. Cambridge MA and London: The Belknap Press of Harvard University Press, 1967.

Bradwell, Stephen. *Physick for the Sicknesse, Commonly called the Plague.* London: Benjamin Fisher, 1636. *Early English Books Online.* 3 March 2008.

Broad, Jacqueline. "Cavendish, Van Helmont, and the Mad Raging Womb." *The New Science and Women's Literary Discourse: Prefiguring Frankenstein.* Ed. Judy A. Hayden. New York: Palgrave Macmillan, 2011. 47–63.

Brown, Ted. "Word Wars: The Debate over the Use of the Vernacular in Medical Writings of the English Renaissance." *Texas Studies in Literature and Language* 37.1 (1995): 98–113. *JSTOR.* 11 August 2015.

Browne, Sir Thomas. *Pseudodoxia Epidemica, or, Enquiries into very many received tenents and commonly presumed truths.* London: T. H. for Edward Dod, 1646. *Early English Books Online.* 22 February 2013.

Religio Medici, Hydriotaphia, and the Letter to a Friend. New York: Scribner, Welford, 1869. Repr. Renascence Editions, 1998. 15 January 2012.

Brugis, Thomas. *The Marrow of Physicke: Or, A learned Discourse of the severall parts of mans Body.* London: Richard Hearne, 1640. *Early English Books Online.* 27 May 2008.

Bulloker, John. *An English Expositor: Teaching the Interpretation of the hardest words used in our Language.* London: J. L., 1654. *Early English Books Online.* 18 February 2012.

Bunworth, Richard: "The Doctresse." *The Doctresse: A Plaine and Easie Method, of Curing Those Disease Which Are Peculiar to Women.* London: J. F. for Nicolas Bourne, 1656. *Early English Books Online.* 3 June 2008.

Burke, Kenneth. *The Rhetoric of Religion: Studies in Logology.* Berkeley: University of California Press, 1970.

Burton, Gideon O. *Silva Rhetoricæ: The Forest of Rhetoric.* 2007. Online resource.

Calvert, Thomas. *Heartsalve for a Wounded Soule. Or, Meditations of comfort for relief of a Soule sick of delayed prayers, and the hiding of Gods countenance.* London: Thomas Broad, 1647. *Early English Books Online.* 16 October 2013.

Capp, Bernard. "Coelson, Lancelot (1627–1687?)." *Oxford Dictionary of National Biography.* Oxford University Press, 2004. 8 August 2013.

"carneous, adj.". *OED Online.* September 2013. Oxford University Press. 24 October 2013.

Cary, Walter. *A Breefe Treatise, Called Caryes Farewell to Physicke*. London: Henrie Denham, 1587. *Early English Books Online*. 27 May 2008.

Castle, George. *The Chymical Galenist*. London: Sarah Griffin, 1667. *Early English Books Online*. 9 September 2010.

Chamberlayne, Thomas. *The Compleat Midwife's Practice Enlarged*. 2nd edn. Cornhill: Nath. Brook, 1659. *Early English Books Online*. 16 October 2013.

Churchill, Wendy D. *Female Patients in Early Modern Britain: Gender, Diagnosis, and Treatment*. Farnham, UK, and Burlington, VT: Ashgate, 2013.

Clarke, Elizabeth. "Ejaculation or Virgin Birth?: The Gendering of the Religious Lyric in the Interregnum." *"This Double Voice": Gendered Writing in Early Modern England*. Ed. Danielle Clarke and Elizabeth Clarke. New York: St. Martin's Press, 2000. 208–29.

Clarke, Samuel. *Medulla theologiae, or, The marrow of divinity contained in sundry questions and cases of conscience, both speculative and practical*. London: Thomas Ratcliff, 1659. *Early English Books Online*. 16 October 2013.

Clericuzio, Antonio. "From van Helmont to Boyle: A Study of the Transmission of Helmontian Chemical and Medical Theories in Seventeenth-Century England." *The British Journal for the History of Science* 26.3 (1993): 303–34. *JSTOR*. 1 October 2013.

Cock, Thomas. *Kitchin-Physick: Or Advice to the Poor, by Way of Dialogue*. London: J. B., 1675. *Early English Books Online*. 3 June 2008.

Miscelanea Medica: Or, A Supplement ot Kitchin-Physick. London, 1675. *Early English Books Online*. 31 May 2008.

Coelson, Lancelot. *The Poor-Mans Physician and Cyrurgion*.London: A. M. for Simon Miller, 1656. *Early English Books Online*. 27 May 2008.

Collins, An. *Divine Songs and Meditacions* (1653). Ed. Sidney Gottlieb. Tempe, AZ: Medieval and Renaissance Texts & Studies, 1996.

Considine, John. "Grey, Elizabeth, Countess of Kent (1582–1651)." *Oxford Dictionary of National Biography*, Oxford: Oxford University Press, 2006. 26 May 2013.

Cook, Harold J. "Bonham, Thomas (c.1564–c.1628)." *Oxford Dictionary of National Biography*. Oxford: Oxford University Press, 2004. 8 March 2013.

The Decline of the Old Medical Regime in Stuart London. Ithaca, NY, and London: Cornell University Press, 1986.

"Good Advice and Little Medicine: The Professional Authority of Early Modern English Physicians." *The Journal of British Studies* 33.1 (1994): 1–31. *JSTOR*. 16 June 2010.

"Victories for Empiricism, Failures for Theory: Medicine and Science in the Seventeenth Century." *The Body as Object and Instrument of Knowledge: Embodied Empiricism in Early Modern Science*. Ed. C. T. Wolfe and O. Gal. *Studies in History and Philosophy of Science* 25. Springer, 2010. 9–31. Ebook.

Cooley, Ronald W. *"Full of All Knowledg": George Herbert's "Country Parson" and Early Modern Social Discourse*.Toronto: University of Toronto Press, 2004.

Coulehan, John L. "The Word Is an Instrument of Healing." *Literature and Medicine* 10 (1991): 111–29. *ProQuest*. 29 July 2008.

Cotta, John. *A Short Discoverie of the Unobserved Dangers of Severall Sorts of Ignorant and Unconsiderate Practisers of Physicke in England.* London: William Jones, 1612. *Early English Books Online.* 18 July 2008.

Crawford, Patricia. "Printed Advertisements for Women Medical Practitioners in London, 1670–1710." *Society for the Social History of Medicine Bulletin* 35 (1984): 66–70.

Cressy, David. "Literacy in Seventeenth-Century England: More Evidence." *The Journal of Interdisciplinary History* 8.1 (1977): 141–50. *JSTOR.* 15 October 2013.

Cummins, Juliet and David Burchell. "Introduction: Ways of Knowing: Conversations between Science, Literature, and Rhetoric." *Science, Literature and Rhetoric in Early Modern England.* Aldershot, UK, and Burlington, VT: Ashgate, 2007. 1–12.

Curry, Patrick. "Culpeper, Nicholas (1616–1654)." *Oxford Dictionary of National Biography.* Oxford: Oxford University Press, 2004. 8 March 2013.

Dickson, Donald R. "Henry Vaughan as Country Doctor." *Explorations in Renaissance Culture* 33.2 (2007): 171–95.

"Henry Vaughan's Medical Annotations." *The Huntington Library Quarterly* 70.3 (2007): 427–52. *ProQuest.* 13 March 2012.

DiMeo, Michelle and Sara Pennell. *Reading and Writing Recipe Books, 1550–1800.* Manchester and New York: Manchester University Press, 2013.

"Introduction." In DiMeo and Pennell, 1–22.

Donne, John. *The Complete English Poems.* Ed. A. J. Smith. London and New York: Penguin, 1971.

Devotions Upon Emergent Occasions. Blackmask Online, 2002. 2 May 2012.

Duffin, Jacalyn. "The Doctor Was Surprised; or, How to Diagnose a Miracle." *Bulletin of the History of Medicine* 81 (2007): 699–729. *Project Muse.* 17 June 2009.

Dunton, John. *The House of Weeping: Or, Mans Last Progress to His Long Home.* London: Black Raven, 1682. *Early English Books Online.* 13 February 2015.

Eberwein, Jane Donahue. "'No Rhet'ric We Expect': Argumentation in Bradstreet's 'The Prologue'." *Early American Literature* 16.1 (1981): 19–26. *JSTOR.* 6 November 2009.

Edwards, Edward. *The Analysis of Chyrurgery: Being the Theorique and Practique part thereof.* London: Thomas Harper, 1636. *Early English Books Online.* 18 July 2008.

The Cure of All Sorts of Fevers. London: Thomas Harper, 1638. *Early English Books Online.* 18 July 2008.

"Eliza." *Eliza's Babes: Or the Virgin's Offering.* London: M. S. for Laurence Blaiklock, 1652. *Early English Books Online.* 4 December 2011.

Elmer, Peter. "*Cotta, John: A Short Discoverie* (1575?–1627/8)." *Oxford Dictionary of National Biography.* Oxford: Oxford University Press, 2004. 8 March 2013.

"Medicine, Religion and the Puritan Revolution." *The Medical Revolution of the Seventeenth Century.* Ed. Roger French and Andrew Wear. Cambridge: Cambridge University Press, 1989. 10–45.

"Medicine, Witchcraft and the Politics of Healing in Late-Seventeenth-Century England." *Medicine and Religion in Enlightenment Europe.* Ed. Ole Peter Grell and Andrew Cunningham. Aldershot, UK, and Burlington, VT: Ashgate, 2007. 223–41.

English, Peter. "Comment on the First Book." *Galen's Method of Physick*. Trans. Peter English. London: A. A. for George Suintoun and James Glen, 1656. 13–18. *Early English Books Online*. 4 December 2011.

Ezell, Margaret J. M. "Cooking the Books, Or, The Three Faces of Hannah Woolley." In DiMeo and Pennell, 159–78.

"Ann Halkett's Morning Devotions: Posthumous Publication and the Culture of Writing in Late Seventeenth-Century Britain." *Print, Manuscript & Performance*. Ed. Arthur F. Marotti and Michael D. Bristol. Columbus: Ohio State University Press, 2000. 215–31.

Enssle, Neal. "Patterns of Godly Life: The Ideal Parish Minister in Sixteenth- and Seventeenth-Century English Thought." *The Sixteenth Century Journal* 28.1 (1997): 3–28. 16 June 2010.

Farrell, Thomas B. "Narrative in Natural Discourse: On Conversation and Rhetoric." *Journal of Communication* (Autumn 1985): 109–27.

"febris, n.". *OED Online*. September 2013. Oxford University Press. 24 October 2013.

Fenner, William. *Practicall divinitie: or, gospel-light shining forth in severall choyce sermons, on divers texts of scripture*. London: T. R. and E. M. for John Stafford, 1647. *Early English Books Online*. 21 October 2013.

Field, Catherine. "'Many hands hands': Writing the Self in Early Modern Women's Recipe Books." *Genre and Womens' Life Writing in Early Modern England*. Ed. Michelle M. Dowd and Julie A. Eckerle. Farnham, UK, and Burlington, VT: Ashgate, 2007: 49–64. 29 October 2013.

Findley, Sandra and Elaine Hobby. "Seventeenth Century Women's Autobiography." *1642: Literature and Power in the Seventeenth Century*. Ed. Francis Barker, Jay Bernstein, John Coombes, Peter Hulme, Jennifer Stone, and Jon Stratton. Colchester, UK: University of Essex Press, 1980. 11–36.

Fish, Stanley E. *Self-Consuming Artifacts: The Experience of Seventeenth-Century Literature*. Berkeley: University of California Press, 1972.

Fissell, Mary E. "Introduction: Women, Health, and Healing in Early Modern Europe." *Bulletin of the History of Medicine* 82.1 (2008): 1–17. *Project Muse*. 11 August 2015.

"The Marketplace of Print." *Medicine and the Market in England and Its Colonies*. Ed. Mark S. R. Jenner and Patrick Wallis. Basingstoke, UK: Palgrave Macmillan, 2007. 108–32.

Fonteyn, Nicolas. *The Womans Doctor: Or, an exact and distinct explantion of all such diseases as are peculiar to that sex with choise and experiementall remedies against the same*. London: John Blague and Samuel Howes, 1652. *Early English Books Online*. 4 December 2011.

Fortuna, Stefania. "Galen's *De Constitutione Artis Medicae* in the Renaissance." *The Classical Quarterly, New Series* 43.1 (1993): 302–19. *JSTOR*. 21 October 2013.

Foucault, Michel. *The Birth of the Clinic: An Archaeology of Medical Perception*. Trans. A. M. Sheridan. London and New York: Routledge, 1989. Kindle file.

Foxley, Rachel. "'The Wildernesse of Tropes and Figures': Figuring Rhetoric in Leveller Pamphlets." *Seventeenth Century* 21.2 (2006): 270–86.

Frank, Arthur W. "The Rhetoric of Self-Change: Illness Experience as Narrative." *The Sociological Quarterly* 34.1 (1993): 39–52. *JSTOR.* 29 July 2008.

Freidson, Eliot. *Profession of Medicine: A Study of the Sociology of Applied Knowledge.* New York: Dodd, Mead, 1973.

Fuller, Thomas. *The Cause and Cure of a Wounded Conscience.*London: G. D. for John Williams, 1649. *Early English Books Online.* 21 October 2013.

Furdell, Elizabeth Lane. *Publishing and Medicine in Early Modern England.* Rochester, NY: University of Rochester Press, 2002.

Galen. *Certaine Workes of Galens, called Methodus Medendi.* Trans. Thomas Gale. London, 1586. *Early English Books Online.* 12 July 2010.

Galen's Method of Physick. Trans. Peter English. London: A. A. for George Suintoun and James Glen, 1656. *Early English Books Online.* December 2011.

Gallagher, Michael P. "Rhetoric, Style, and George Herbert." *ELH* 37.4 (1970): 495–516.

Garden, Rebecca. "The Problem of Empathy: Medicine and the Humanities." *New Literary History* 38.3 (2007): 551–67. *Project Muse.* 7 July 2010.

"Telling Stories about Illness and Disability: The Limits and Lessons of Narrative." *Perspectives in Biology and Medicine* 53.1 (2010): 121–35. *Project Muse.* 7 July 2010.

Gatford, Lionell. *Logos Alexipharmakos: or, Hyperphysicall Directions in Time of Plague.* Oxford: H. Hall, 1644. *Early English Books Online.* 18 July 2008.

Gevitz, Norman. " 'The Devil Hath Laughed at the Physicians': Witchcraft and Medical Practice in Seventeenth-Century New England." *Journal of the History of Medicine and Allied Sciences* 55.1 (2000): 5–36.

Gibson, Joan. "Educating for Silence: Renaissance Women and the Language Arts." *Hyptatia* 4.1 (1989): 9–27.

Gillett, Grant. "Virtue and Truth in Clincal Science." *The Journal of Medicine and Philopsophy* 20 (1995): 285–98.

Godfrey, Robert. *Various Injuries & Abuses in Chymical and Galenical Physick.* London: John Darby for Richard Jones, 1674. *Early English Books Online.* 9 July 2010.

Goldberg, Jonathan. "The Understanding of Sickness in Donne's Devotions." *Renaissance Quarterly* 24.4 (1971): 507–17. *JSTOR.* 16 June 2010.

Goldstein, Jan. "Foucault among the Sociologists: The 'Disciplines' and the History of the Professions." *History and Theory* 23.2 (1984): 170–192. *JSTOR.* 1 October 2013.

Gottlieb, Sidney. "An Collins and the Experience of Defeat." *Representing Women in Renaissance England.* Ed. Claude J. Summers and Ted-Larry Pebworth. Columbia, MO: University of Missouri Press, 1997. 216–26.

Gouk, Penelope. "Performance Practice: Music, Medicine and Natural Philosophy in Interregnum Oxford." *The British Journal for the History of Science* 29.3 (1996): 257–88. *JSTOR.* 25 July 2013.

Gowland, Angus. *The Worlds of Renaissance Melancholy: Robert Burton in Context.* Cambridge: Cambridge University Press, 2006.

Green, Monica H. *Making Women's Medicine Masculine: The Rise of Male Authority in Pre-Modern Gynaecology.* Oxford: Oxford University Press, 2008.

Greene, Thomas M. *The Light in Troy: Imitation and Discovery in Renaissance Poetry*. New Haven, CT: Yale University Press, 1982.

Grey, Elizabeth. *A Choice Manual of Rare and Select Secrets in Physick and Cyrurgery*. London: W. I., 1653. *Early English Books Online*. 18 July 2008.

Griffin, Andrew. "John Banister (1532/3–1599?)." *Oxford Dictionary of National Biography*. Ed. H. C. G. Matthew and Brian Harrison. Oxford: Oxford University Press, 2004. Online edn. Ed. Lawrence Goldman. Oct. 2008. 8 May 2013.

Halkett, Lady Anne. *The Autobiography of Anne, Lady Halkett*. Ed. John Gough Nichols. Westminster, UK: Camden Society, 1875.

Hammond, Henry. *A paraphrase & annotations upon the Psalms*. 1659. Repr. *The works of the reverend and learned Henry Hammond, D. D.* London: T. Newcomb and M. Flesher, 1684. *Early English Books Online*. 21 October 2013.

Harley, David. "James Hart of Northampton and the Calvinist Critique of Priest-Physicians: An Unpublished Polemic of the Early 1620s." *Medical History* 42 (1998): 362–86.

"Rhetoric and the Social Construction of Illness and Healing." *Social History of Medicine* 12.3 (1999): 407–35.

Hart, James. *A Discourse of the lawless intrusion of Parsons & vicars upon the profession of Physicke with the absurditie of the same*. Bodleian Library: MS. Rawl. D. 146.

KJIINIKH, or the Diet of the Diseased. London: John Beale, 1633. *Early English Books Online*. 18 July 2008.

Hartill, Graham. "'Healing Wings': Henry Vaughan and the Poetics of Healing." *Scintilla* 1 (1997): 9–19.

Healy, Margaret. "'Seeing' Contagious Bodies in Early Modern London." *The Body in Late Medieval and Early Modern Culture*.Ed. Darryll Grantley and Nina Taunton. Burlington, VT, and Aldershot, UK: Ashgate, 2000. 157–68.

Henry, John. "The Matter of Souls: Medical Theory and Theology in Seventeenth-Century England." *The Medical Revolution of the Seventeenth Century*. Ed. Roger French and Andrew Wear. Cambridge: Cambridge University Press, 1989. 87–113.

Hensley, Jeannine. "A Note on the Text." *The Works of Anne Bradstreet*. Ed. Jeannine Hensley. Cambridge MA: Belknap/Harvard University Press, 1967. xxxvii–xxxviii.

Herbert, George. *A Priest to the Temple: Or, The Country Parson, His Character, and Rule of Holy Life*. In *George Herbert: The Complete English Poems*. Ed. John Tobin. London, New York, and Toronto: Penguin, 1991. 199–263.

Heron, Edward. *Physicke for Body and Soule. Shewing that the Maladies of the one, proceede from the sinnes of the other*. London: John Legatt for Francis Constable, 1621. *Early English Books Online*. 18 July 2008.

Hildebrand, Anne. "Anne Bradstreet's Quaternions and 'Contemplations'." *Early American Literature* 8.2 (1973): 117–25. *JSTOR*. 12 June 2012.

Hinds, Hilary. *God's Englishwomen: Seventeenth-Century Radical Sectarian Writing and Feminist Criticism*. Manchester and New York: Manchester University Press, 1996.

Hobbes, Thomas. *The Art of Rhetoric, with A Discourse of the Laws of England.* London: William Crooke, 1681. *Early English Books Online.* 21 August 2008.

Hobby, Elaine. "Notes." *The Midwives Book* by Jane Sharp. Oxford: Oxford UP, 1999.

Hodgkins, Christopher. "'Showing Holy': Herbert and the Rhetoric of Sincerity." *New Perspectives on the Seventeenth Century English Religious Lyric.* Ed. John R. Roberts. Columbia: University of Missouri Press, 1993. 222–36.

Horobin, Gordon. "Professional Mystery: The Maintenance of Charisma in General Medical Practice." *The Sociology of the Professions: Lawyers, Doctors and Others.* Ed. Robert Dingwall and Philip Lewis. New York: St. Martin's Press, 1983. 84–105.

Huebert, Ronald. "The Private Opinions of Sir Thomas Browne." *SEL: Studies in English Literature, 1500–1900* 45.1 (2005): 117–134. *JSTOR.* 30 January 2012.

Hunter, Jeanne Clayton. "George Herbert and Puritan Piety." *The Journal of Religion* 68.2 (1988): 226–41. *JSTOR.* 21 October 2013.

Hunter, Lynette. "Women and Domestic Medicine: Lady Experimenters, 1570–1620." *Women, Science and Medicine 1500–1700.* Ed. Lynette Hunter and Sarah Hutton. Phoenix Mill, UK: Sutton, 1997. 89–107.

Hunter, Lynette and Sarah Hutton. "Women, Science and Medicine: Introduction." In *Women, Science and Medicine 1500–1700.* Ed. Lynette Hunter and Sarah Hutton. Phoenix Mill, UK: Sutton, 1997. 1–6.

Hurley, Ann. "An Collins: The Tradition of the Religious Lyric, Modified or Corrected?" *Discovering and (Re)Covering the Seventeenth Century Religious Lyric.* Ed. Eugene R. Cunnar and Jeffrey Johnson. Pittsburgh: Duquesne University Press, 2001. 231–47.

"implexure, n.". *OED Online.* September 2013. Oxford University Press. 28 October 2013.

Innocenti, Beth. "A Normative Pragmatic Model of Making Fear Appeals." *Philosophy and Rhetoric* 44.3 (2011): 273–290. *Project Muse.* 17 July 2012.

Jenner, Mark S. R. and Patrick Wallis. "The Medical Marketplace." *Medicine and the Market in England and Its Colonies.* Ed. Mark S. R. Jenner and Patrick Wallis. Basingstoke, UK: Palgrave Macmillan, 2007. 1–23.

Johnson, Bruce A. "The Audience Shift in George Herbert's Poetry." *SEL: Studies in English Literature, 1500–1900* 35.1 (1995): 89–103. *JSTOR.* 20 February 2013.

Johnson, T. R. "Writing as Healing and the Rhetorical Tradition: Sorting Out Plato, Postmodernism, Writing Pedagogy, and Post-Traumatic Stress Disorder." *Writing and Healing: Toward an Informed Practice.* Ed. Charles M. Anderson and Marian M. MacCurdy. Urbana, IL: NCTE Press, 2000. 85–114.

Kearns, Judith. "Fashioning Innocence: Rhetorical Construction of Character in the Memoirs of Anne, Lady Halkett." *Texas Studies in Literature and Language* 46.3 (2004): 340–62.

Keller, Eve. "Mrs Jane Sharp: Midwifery and the Critique of Medical Knowledge in Seventeenth-Century England." *Women's Writing* 2.2 (1995): 101–11.

Kelly, Louis G. "London Apothecaries as Early Christians: Renewing the Covenant." *Healing in Religion and Society, from Hippocrates to the Puritans.*

Ed. J. Kevin Coyle and Steven C. Muir. Lewiston, NY: The Edwin Mellen Press, 1999. 159–86.

Kerwin, William. "Where Have You Gone, Margaret Kennix? Seeking the Tradition of Healing Women in English Renaissance Drama." *Women Healers and Physicians: Climbing a Long Hill.* Ed. Lilian R. Furst. Lexington: The University Press of Kentucky, 1997. 93–113.

Kirmayer, Laurence J. "The Body's Insistence on Meaning: Metaphor as Presentation and Representation in Illness Experience." *Medical Anthropology Quarterly* 6.4 (1992): 323–46. *JSTOR.* 12 March 2013.

Knight, Katherine. "A Precious Medicine: Tradition and Magic in Some Seventeenth-Century Household Remedies." *Folklore* 113.2 (2002): 237–47. *JSTOR.* 15 March 2013.

Knoppers, Laura Lunger. "Opening the Queen's Closet: Henrietta Maria, Elizabeth Cromwell, and the Politics of Cookery." *Renaissance Quarterly* 60.2 (2007): 464–99. *JSTOR.* 24 August 2015.

Laín Entralgo, Pedro. *The Therapy of the Word in Classical Antiquity.* 1958. Ed. and Trans. L. J. Rather and John M. Sharp. New Haven, CT, and London: Yale University Press, 1970.

Lamb, Mary Ellen. "Merging the Secular and the Spiritual in Lady Anne Halkett's Memoirs." *Genre and Women's Life Writing in Early Modern England.* Ed. Michelle M. Dowd and Julie A. Eckerle. Aldershot, UK, and Burlington, VT: Ashgate, 2007. 81–96.

Lander, Clara. "A Dangerous Sickness Which Turned to a Spotted Fever." *SEL: Studies in English Literature, 1500–1900* 11.1 (1971): 89–108. *JSTOR.* 17 June 2010.

Lanham, Richard. *A Handlist of Rhetorical Terms.* 2nd edn. Berkeley: University of California Press, 1991.

Laroche, Rebecca. *Medical Authority and Englishwomen's Herbal Texts, 1550–1650.* Farnham, UK, and Burlington, VT: Ashgate, 2009.

LeJacq, Seth Stein. "The Bounds of Domestic Healing: Medical Recipes, Storytelling and Surgery in Early Modern England." *Social History of Medicine* 26.3 (2013): 451–68. *Oxford Journals.* 11 August 2015.

Leong, Elaine. "Collecting Knowledge for the Family: Recipes, Gender and Practical Knowledge in the Early Modern English Household." *Centaurus* 55 (2013): 81–103.

"'Herbals she peruseth': Reading Medicine in Early modern England." *Renaissance Studies* 28.4 (2014): 556–78.

Linden, Stanton J. "Mrs. Mary Trye, Medicatrix: Chemistry and Controversy in Restoration England." *Women's Writing* 1.3 (1994): 341–53.

Lingo, Alison Klairmont. "Empirics and Charlatans in Early Modern France: The Genesis of the Classification of the 'Other' in Medical Practice. "*Journal of Social History* 19.4 (1986): 583–603. *JSTOR.* 13 August 2008.

Lutes, Jean Marie. "Negotiating Theology and Gynecology: Anne Bradstreet's Representations of the Female Body." *Signs* 22.2 (1997): 309–40. *JSTOR.* 11 June 2009.

M., A. *A Rich Closet of Physical Secrets*. London: Gartrude Dawson, 1652. *Early English Books Online*. 27 May 2008.

MacDonald, Keith M. *The Sociology of the Professions*. London and Thousand Oaks, CA: Sage, 1995.

Mack, Phyllis. *Visionary Women: Ecstatic Prophecy in Seventeenth-Century England*. Berkeley: University of California Press, 1992.

Mack, Peter. "Rhetoric, Ethics and Reading in the Renaissance." *Renaissance Studies* 19.1 (2005): 1–21.

Maclean, Ian. "The 'Sceptical Crisis' Reconsidered: Galen, Rational Medicine and the *Libertas Philosophandi*. *Early Science and Medicine* 11.3 (2006): 247–74. *JSTOR*. 21 October 2013.

Magee, Reginald. "Medical Practice and Medical Education 1500–2001: An Overview." *ANZ Journal of Surgery* 74 (2004): 272–76.

Magro, Maria. "Spiritual Autobiography and Radical Sectarian Women's Discourse: Anna Trapnel and the Bad Girls of the English Revolution." *Journal of Medieval and Early Modern Studies* 34.2 (2004): 405–37. *Project Muse*. 18 August 2009.

Malcolmson, Cristina. "George Herbert's 'Country Parson' and the Character of Social Identity." *Studies in Philology* 85.2 (1988): 245–66. 16 June 2010.

Mann, Jenny C. *Figuring Vernacular Eloquence in Shakespeare's England*. Ithaca, NY: Cornell University Press, 2012.

Margerum, Eileen. "Anne Bradstreet's Public Poetry and the Tradition of Humility." *Early American Literature* 17.2 (1982): 152–60. *JSTOR*. 30 May 2012.

Markham, Gervase. *The English House-Wife*. London: Nicholas Okes, 1631. *Early English Books Online*. 18 July 2008.

McConchie, R. W. "Additions to *OED* from John Cotta's *Ignorant Practisers of Physicke*, 1612." *Notes and Queries* 28.6 (1981): 490–93. 30 May 2013.

McElligott, Jason. "Gatford, Lionel (*d.* 1665)." *Oxford Dictionary of National Biography*. Oxford University Press, 2004. 25 July 2013.

Merret, Christopher. *The Accomplisht Physician, the Honest Apothecary, and the Skilful Chyrurgeon*.London, 1670. *Early English Books Online*. 9 July 2010.

Milton, John. *Areopagitica*. 1644. Renascence Editions, 2005. 28 August 2012.

Morrissey, Thomas J. "The Self and the Meditative Tradition in Donne's 'Devotions'." *Notre Dame English Journal* 13.1 (1980): 29–49. *JSTOR*. 15 January 2012.

Narveson, Kate. "Flesh, Excrement, Humors, Nothing: The Body in Early Stuart Devotional Discourse." *Studies in Philology* 96.3 (1999): 313–33. 17 June 2010.

Papazian, Mary Arshagouni. "Donne, Election, and the 'Devotions upon Emergent Occasions.'" *Huntington Library Quarterly* 55.4 (1992): 603–19. *JSTOR*. 17 June 2010.

Paracelsus. *Of Chymical Transmutation*.Trans. R. Turner. London: Richard Moon and Henry Fletcher, 1657. *Early English Books Online*. 2 January 2012.

Peacham, Henry. *The Garden of Eloquence*. London: R. F. for H. Jackson, 1593. *Early English Books Online*. 21 August 2008.

Pearcy, Lee T. "Diagnosis as Narrative in Ancient Literature." *The American Journal of Philology* 113.4 (1992): 595–616. *JSTOR*. 9 July 2010.

Pelling, Margaret. *Medical Conflicts in Early Modern London: Patronage, Physicians, and Irregular Practitioners, 1550–1640*. Oxford: Oxford University Press, 2003.

"Trade or Profession?: Medical Practice in Early Modern England." *The Common Lot: Sickness, Medical Occupations, and the Urban Poor in Early Modern England*. London: Longman, 1998. 230–58.

Pelling, Margaret and Charles Webster. "Medical Practitioners." *Health, Medicine, and Mortality in the Sixteenth Century*. Ed. Charles Webster. Cambridge: Cambridge University Press, 1979. 165–235.

Pender, Patricia. *Early Modern Women's Writing and the Rhetoric of Modesty*. Basingstoke, UK: Palgrave Macmillan, 2012.

Pender, Stephen. "Between Medicine and Rhetoric." *Early Science and Medicine* 10.1 (2005): 36–64.

"Essaying the Body: Donne, Affliction, and Medicine." *John Donne's Professional Lives*. Ed. David Colclough. Cambridge: DS Brewer, 2003. 215–48.

"Examples and Experience: On the Uncertainty of Medicine." *The British Journal for the History of Science*, 39.1 (2006): 1–28. *JSTOR*. 15 January 2012.

"Rhetoric, Grief, and the Imagination in Early Modern England." *Philosophy and Rhetoric* 43.1 (2010): 54–85.

"Signs of Interiority, or Epistemology in the Bodyshop." *The Dalhousie Review* 85.2 (2005): 221–37.

"Subventing Disease: Anger, Passions, and the Non-Naturals." *Rhetorics of Bodily Disease and Health in Medieval and Early Modern England*. Ed. Jennifer C. Vaught. Aldershot, UK, and Burlington, VT: Ashgate, 2012. 193–218.

Pennebaker, James. "Telling Stories: The Health Benefits of Narrative." *Literature and Medicine* 19.1 (2000): 3–18.

"phthisis, n.". *OED Online*. September 2013. Oxford University Press. 24 October 2013.

Pickstone, John V. "Working Knowledges before and after circa 1800: Practices and Disciplines in the History of Science, Technology, and Medicine." *Isis* 98.3 (2007): 489–516. *JSTOR*. 15 March 2013.

"pinguid, adj.". *OED Online*. September 2013. Oxford University Press. 24 October 2013.

Plato, *Phaedrus*. Trans. Benjamin Jowett. The Gutenberg Project. 19 March 2013.

Pollock, Linda. *With Faith and Physic: The Life of a Tudor Gentlewoman, Lady Grace Mildmay 1552–1620*. London: Collins & Brown, 1993.

Porter, Roy. *Bodies Politic: Disease, Death and Doctors in Britain, 1650–1900*. Ithaca, NY: Cornell University Press, 2001.

"The Patient's View: Doing Medical History from Below." *Theory and Society* 14.2 (1985): 175–98. *JSTOR*. 29 July 2008.

Prideaux, John. *Sacred Eloquence: Or, the Art of Rhetorick, As it is layd down in Scripture*. London: W. Wilson, 1659. *Early English Books Online*. 23 March 2013.

Primrose, James. *Popular Errours: or, the Errours of the People in Physick*.Trans. Robert Witty. London: W. Wilson, 1651. *Early English Books Online*. 4 December 2011.

Purkiss, Diane. "Producing the Voice, Consuming the Body: Women Prophets of the Seventeenth Century." *Women, Writing, History 1640–1740*. Ed. Isobel Grundy and Susan Wiseman. London: B. T. Batsford, 1992. 139–58.

Ramus, Petrus. *A Compendium of the Art of Logic and Rhetorick*. London: Thomas Maxey, 1651. *Early English Books Online*. 21 August 2008.

Raymond, Joad. "Nedham, Marchamont (bap. 1620, d. 1678)." *Oxford Dictionary of National Biography*. Oxford: Oxford University Press, 2004. 26 May 2013.

Rex, Michael. "Eyes on the Prize: The Search for Personal Space and Stability through Religious Devotion in *Eliza's Babes*." *Discovering and (Re)Covering the Seventeenth Century Religious Lyric*. Ed. Eugene R. Cunnar and Jeffrey Johnson. Pittsburgh: Duquesne University Press, 2001. 205–30.

Rogers, Timothy. *Practical Discourse on Sickness & Recovery in Several Sermons*. London: Thomas Parkhurst, 1691. *Early English Books Online*. 21 March 2013.

Rose, Hilary. "Foreword: From Household to Public Knowledge, to a New Production System of Knowledge." In *Women, Science and Medicine 1500–1700*. Ed. Lynette Hunter and Sarah Hutton. Phoenix Mill, UK: Sutton, 1997. xi–xx.

Sadler, John. *The Sick Womans Private Looking-Glasse*. London: Philip Stephens and Charles Meredith, 1636. *Early English Books Online*. 4 December 2011.

Scarry, Elaine. *The Body in Pain: The Making and Unmaking of the World*. New York: Oxford University Press, 1985.

Scudder, Henry. *The Christians Daily Walke in Holy Securitie and Peace*. London: J. B. for Henry Overton, 1631. *Early English Books Online*. 26 March 2013.

Segal, Judy Z. "Illness as Argumentation: A Prolegomenon to the Rhetorical Study of Contestable Complaints." *Health: An Interdisciplinary Journal for the Social Study of Health, Illness and Medicine* 11. 2 (2007): 227–44. 16 August 2009.

Selleck, Nancy. "Donne's Body." *SEL: Studies in English Literature, 1500–1900* 41.1 (2001): 149–74. *JSTOR*. 6 September 2009.

Semler, L. E. "Textual Notes and Commentary." *Eliza's Babes: Or the Virgin's Offering 1652, a Critical Edition*. Ed. L. E. Semler. London: Associated University Press, 2001. 139–94.

Shapiro, Barbara J. "Law and Science in Seventeenth-Century England." *Stanford Law Review* 21.4 (1969): 727–66. *JSTOR*. 1 October 2013.

Sharp, Jane. *The Midwives Book*. London: Simon Miller, 1671. *Women Writers Online*. 4 December 2011.

Shaw, A. Batty. "Sir Thomas Browne: The Man and the Physician." *British Medical Journal* (Clinical Research Edition) 285.6334 (1982): 40–42. *JSTOR*. 30 January 2012.

Shaw, Jane. "Fasting Women: The Significance of Gender and Bodies in Radical Religion and Politics, 1650–1813." *Radicalism in British Literary Culture, 1650–1830: From Revolution to Revolution*. Ed. Timothy Morton and Nigel Smith. Cambridge: Cambridge University Press, 2002. 101–15.

Sheridan, Bridgette. "Whither Childbearing: Gender, Status and the Professionalization of Medicine in Early Modern France." *Gender and Scientific Discourse*

in Early Modern Culture. Ed. Kathleen P. Long. Burlington, VT: Ashgate, 2010. 239–58.
Sherwood, Thomas. *The Charitable Pestmaster, Or, the Cure of the Plague*. London: A. N. for John Francklin, 1641. *Early English Books Online*. 9 August 2010.
Sibbes, Richard. *Bowels opened, or, A discovery of the neere and deere love, union and communion betwixt Christ and the Church, and consequently betweixt Him and every believing soule*. London: George Miller, 1639. *Early English Books Online*. 24 October 2013.
Sidney Herbert, Mary. *The Collected Works of Mary Sidney Herbert, Countess of Pembroke*: Volume II: *The Psalmes of David*. Ed. Margaret P. Hannay, Noel J. Kinnamon, and Michael G. Brennan. Oxford: Oxford English Texts, 1998.
Sidney, Sir Philip. *Defence of Poesie*. (1595). Renascence Editions, 1995. 11 April 2005.
Siraisi, Nancy. "Anatomizing the Past: Physicians and History in Renaissance Culture." *Renaissance Quarterly* 53.1 (2000): 1–30. *JSTOR*. 7 July 2010.
"Oratory and Rhetoric in Renaissance Medicine." *Journal of the History of Ideas*. 65.2 (2004): 191–211. *JSTOR*. 15 October 2011.
Skwire, Sarah E. "Women, Writers, Sufferers: Anne Conway and An Collins." *Literature and Medicine* 18.1 (1999): 1–23.
Smith, John. *The Mysterie of Rhetorick Unveil'd*. London: E. T. and R. H., 1673. *Early English Books Online*. 18 July 2013.
Spencer, Jane. "Creating the Woman Writer: The Autobiographical Works of Jane Barker." *Tulsa Studies in Women's Literature* 2.2 (1983): 165–81. *JSTOR*. 14 March 2012.
Stock, Brian. "Minds, Bodies, Readers." *New Literary History* 37 (2006): 489–501. *Project Muse*. 6 June 2010.
Stolberg, Michael. *Experiencing Illness and the Sick Body in Early Modern Europe*. Basingstoke, UK: Palgrave Macmillan, 2011.
Struever, Nancy. "Petrarch's *Invective Contra Medicum*: An Early Confrontation of Rhetoric and Medicine." *MLN* 108.4 (1993): 659–79. 21 August 2008.
Sugg, Richard. *The Smoke of the Soul: Medicine, Physiology and Religion in Early Modern England*. Basingstoke, UK: Palgrave Macmillan, 2013.
Sumich, Christi. *Divine Doctors and Dreadful Distempers: How Practicing Medicine Became a Respectable Profession*. Amsterdam: Rodopi, 2013.
Sutherland, Christine Mason. *The Eloquence of Mary Astell*. Calgary, AB: University of Calgary Press, 2005.
Tannenbaum, Rebecca J. *The Healer's Calling: Women and Medicine in Early New England*. Ithaca, NY, and London: Cornell University Press, 2002.
Taylor, Jeremy. *The Rule and Exercises of Holy Dying*. London: R. R., 1651. *Early English Books Online*. 4 December 2011.
Temkin, Oswei. *Galenism: Rise and Decline of a Medical Philosophy*. Ithaca, NY, and London: Cornell University Press, 1973.
Thomas, Keith. *Religion and the Decline of Magic: Studies in Popular Beliefs in Sixteenth and Seventeenth-Century England*. London, New York, and Toronto: Penguin, 1991. Kindle file.

Thomson, George. *Galeno-pale: Or, A Chymical Trial of the Galenists*. London: R. Wood, 1665. *Early English Books Online*. 4 December 2011.

Trapnel, Anna. *Anna Trapnel's Report and Plea, Or, a Narrative Of her Journey from London into Cornwal, the occasion of it, the Lord's encouragements to it, and signal presence with her in it*. London: Thomas Brewster, 1654. *Early English Books Online*. 26 March 2013.

The cry of a stone. Or A relation of something spoken in Whitehall, by Anna Trapnel, being in the visions of God. London, 1654. *Early English Books Online*. 4 December 2011.

Trye, Mary. *Medicatrix, or the Woman-Physician*. London: T. R. and N. T., 1675. *Early English Books Online*. 30 May 2013.

van Engen, Abram. "Advertising the Domestic: Anne Bradstreet's Sentimental Poetics." *Legacy* 28.1 (2011): 47–68.

van Foreest, Pieter. *The Arraignment of Urines: Wherein Are Set downe the manifold errors and abuses of ignorant Urine-monging Empirikes, cozening Quacksalvers, women-physitians, and the like stuffe*. London: O. Eld for Robert Mylebourne, 1623. *Early English Books Online*. 4 December 2011.

Wall, Wendy. "Our Bodies/Our Texts? Renaissance Women and the Trials of Authorship." *Anxious Power: Reading, Writing, and Ambivlence in Narrative by Women*. Ed. Carol J. Singley and Susan Elizabeth Sweeney. Albany, NY: State University of New York Press, 1993. 51–72.

Wear, Andrew. *Knowledge and Practice in English Medicine, 1550–1680*. Cambridge: Cambridge University Press, 2000.

"Medical Practice in Late Seventeenth- and Early Eighteenth-Century England: Continuity and Union." *The Medical Revolution of the Seventeenth Century*. Ed. Roger French and Andrew Wear. Cambridge: Cambridge University Press, 1989. 294–320.

"The Popularization of Medicine in Early Modern England." *The Popularization of Medicine 1650–1850*. Ed. Roy Porter. London and New York: Routledge, 1992. 17–41.

"Puritan Perceptions of Illness in Seventeenth Century England." *Patients and Practitioners: Lay Perceptions of Medicine in Pre-Industrial Society*. Cambridge: Cambridge University Press, 2003. 55–99.

Weber, A. S. "Women's Early Modern Medical Almanacs in Historical Context." *ELR: English Literary Renaissance* 33.3 (2003): 358–402.

Webster, Charles. *The Great Instauration: Science, Medicine and Reform, 1626–1660*. London: Duckworth, 1975.

Whaley, Leigh. *Women and the Practice of Medical Care in Early Modern Europe, 1400–1800*. Basingstoke, UK: Palgrave Macmillan, 2011.

White, Elizabeth Wade. "The Tenth Muse – A Tercentenary Appraisal of Anne Bradstreet." *The William and Mary Quarterly* 8.3 (1951): 355–77. *JSTOR*. 11 June 2009.

Williamson, Marilyn L. *Raising Their Voices: British Women Writiers, 1650–1750*. Detroit: Wayne State University Press, 1990.

Wilson, Thomas. *The Art of Rhetoric*. 1560. Ed. Peter E. Medine. University Park: Pennsylvania State University Press, 1994.

Wood, Owen. *An Epitomie of the Most Experienced, Excellent and Profitable Secrets appertaining to Physick and Chirurgery*. London: E. C., 1653. *Early English Books Online*. 9 August 2010.

Wootton, David. *Bad Medicine: Doctors Doing Harm Since Hippocrates*. Oxford: Oxford University Press, 2006. Kindle file.

Younge, Richard. *A sovereign antidote against all grief extracted out of the choisest authors, ancient and modern both holy and humane*. London: Thomas Gataker, 1654. *Early English Books Online*. 16 October 2013.

Index